HEALI

CW01573422

The Autobiography of

Albert Byram

ARTHUR H. STOCKWELL LTD.
Elms Court Ilfracombe Devon
Established 1898

First published in Great Britain, 1996

British Library Cataloguing-in-Publication Data.
A catalogue record for this book is available from the British Library.

By the same author:
Self Help and Movement for Rheumatic Sufferers

ISBN 0 7223 3025-1

Printed in Great Britain by
Arthur H. Stockwell Ltd.
Elms Court Ilfracombe
Devon

Grateful thanks go to all my past patients, and to all who helped with this small book; especially The Oldham Evening Chronicle *for all the help they gave me and the three Golden Wedding photographs. Also my thanks go to Miss Emma Jane Foden, fifteen years old, who corrected my poor writing and also processed this book for me.*

CONTENTS

LIST OF ILLUSTRATIONS

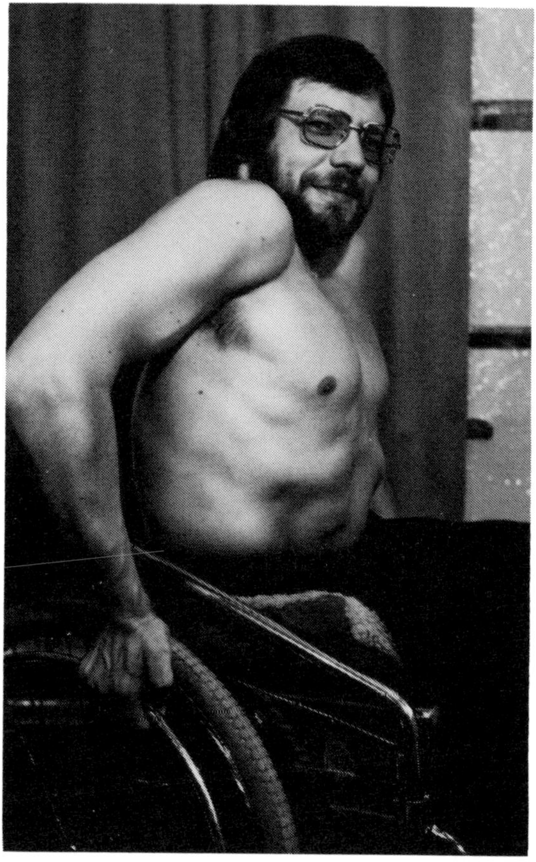

David Foden

FOREWORD

Having been asked to write the foreword to this book, I have pondered long and hard on what I could say in a few words about a man whose full and eventful life could fill an encyclopedia.

I was lucky enough to meet Albert Byram when seven years old and an immediate impact was made. A man who was different, full of self-belief and a true conviction of what was correct and beneficial to others.

Taken under his medical and knowledgeable wing, I have undoubtedly benefited through Mr B, as I affectionately call him. His vast knowledge of not only the human body, but also the human mind, has meant that I am only one of thousands who have had the privilege of receiving those benefits.

"Mr B" has never lost that boy-like sense of fun and mischief, which at times brought concern to Mrs B. However this lovely lady did for her husband the same as every outstanding man has had from his wife, the support of a better woman who loved, cared and provided added strength to the great man.

Mr B carrying me as a boy, and as a young man, on his shoulders laden with fishing tackle across his beloved river, made me believe that nothing was beyond my reach as long as you have the determination and the help of others.

My thanks for enriching my life go to Bert and Nan Byram, a couple the likes of which are fast disappearing from this world, to the detriment of the human race.

Special people should not be forgotten, so may this book offer the opportunity for many more to share these varied, interesting and valuable lives.

David Foden

CHAPTER 1

WARWICK STREET

I was born 11th October 1910, in a poor house with one bedroom and another two rooms downstairs. There was only a front door and in those days we had outdoor toilets, and to get to the toilet we had to go out of Warwick Street (where I lived), down Cambridge Street and then into a cobbled yard where three toilets were shared among eight houses. Our house, which was very old, had flagged floors; in our small kitchen there was a slopstone and also a cellar for coal, that was if we could afford it.

Sometime later we moved next door. The house had two bedrooms and also a back door — this was real luxury to us — we even had a tin bath hung outside on the back wall.

There were four children in my family including myself. My brother Harry died while he was still an infant of tuberculosis; my other brother James had the same and was unable to walk until the age of five. There was then my younger sister Betty; she was a fairly good girl and grew up to be a lovely young lady.

Most people in our area were desperately poor and Cambridge Street was nicknamed Suicide Street as people would hang or gas themselves instead of going to work in the workhouse.

My father worked at Platt Bros., who were known worldwide for the making of cotton spinning machinery. He gained a skilled job and worked twelve hours, from six

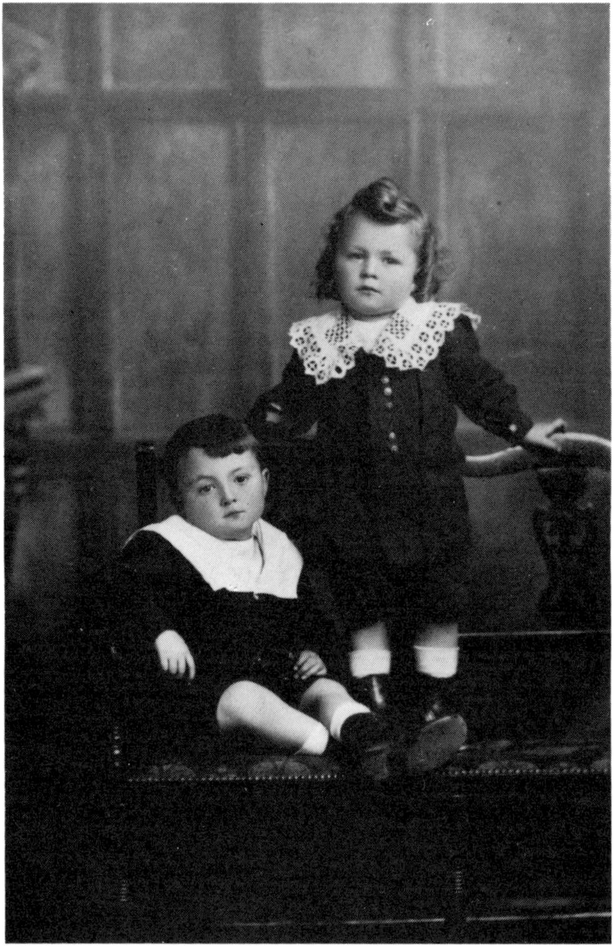

James and Albert Byram (1913)

in the morning till six at night, during the week, and on Saturdays, he would only work from six in the morning till twelve noon. My father was paid eighteen shillings a week. As many other ladies, my mother took in washing to supplement the people who didn't get a good wage.

We managed well until my father joined the Army in 1914 as a Private Soldier, then hunger started to creep in to our family. My mother then had to start work as a Cop Packer in a cotton mill which was situated about a mile away from our house. This was a hard task for Mother with the damp conditions and a lot of bending. Mother also worked for twelve hours a day but, at eight in the morning there was a half an hour break, so Mother used to rush back to us and feed her three hungry children:—James (six and a half), myself (five) and Betty (four).

A couple of years later, we were informed that Father had been badly gassed in France. My mother left us with a kind neighbour, and travelled through London, in an air raid, and managed to see him. My father was unconscious and she did not think that he would live.

Many months later, they brought Dad to Caton Bay, near Scarborough and this time Ma decided that we would all go to see him. She had no spare money, so she bought a railway ticket for only herself. At the railway station we dodged the turnstile and then on the train when the ticket master came round, hid under the seat. At the other end we got away with it again.

Caton Bay was a great thrill, we stayed with the Army but I will always remember that I enjoyed the food at the camp much more than I did at home. Many foods and sugar were rationed, and rice pudding was cooked in a large washing up bowl, and to sweeten it we would put a whole pot of jam in the middle.

One day I remember the great excitement we all had when German ships shelled the castle at Scarborough and our soldiers ran out a small cannon and started to fire. Alas our shells just fell into the sea about a mile from the Jerries.

We had a few weeks' full board with the Army, which we got free, but Dad I am sorry to say was not doing too well. He had hydraemic nephritis and epilepsy and so was transferred to a military hospital.

We then went back home to 60 Warwick Street, which felt colder and damper than ever. Once again on the journey home, us kids travelled free.

CHAPTER 2

WORK

At eight years old I got an evening job, lathering stubby chins, so that the barber could use his cutthroat razor to shave lots of, mostly dirty chins. On Armistice Day, 1918, the excitement was great and everyone was on holiday, but not me; the old barber came for me to go to work. Trade was good all day because people wanted to feel clean shaven to celebrate; I had to lather and like it. I often missed school because I was needed at home or at work earning some money.

One day I had no food so I decided to go to Oldham Market to find the scraps of food that had dropped off the stalls.

Sometime later I got a good evening job that I enjoyed — cleaning Borough Superior motorcycles. I loved these machines and put my all in to the job. My polishing was done with great enthusiasm and I also got paid one shilling and sixpence for each bike that I did. It was possible to polish two bikes in one night which meant even more money. Unfortunately this job was only two nights a week, so I got a paper round for the mornings. I then later sold Saturday Sports papers, the Sunday papers and *Green Final* on the streets.

I enjoyed working as a paperboy but had to dodge the School Board Officer, who was often out looking for underage paperboys, by jumping over walls and dashing through gardens. I was luckily never caught.

CHAPTER 3

1920 — DAD AT HOME

Father came home in 1920, but the epileptic fits gave us great concern. When Father had a fit, the first thing we had to do was to try to squeeze a piece of rubber in between his teeth to stop him from biting right through his tongue. After the terrible convulsions, he would lose consciousness and snore loudly, often for as long as an hour. It may appear strange today that we never sent for a doctor, but as we were poor we had no phone and no money to pay his bill when he came. There was no National Health in those days and it was many years before the doctor had seen Dad having a fit.

Around this time, poor overworked Mother developed rheumatoid arthritis and we were forced to get medical help. A doctor brought an injection, which we were told had come all the way from Germany, and injected it into her hip. A while after Mother had been given the injection an enormous lump came up at the top of her leg. A few weeks later all Ma's teeth became very loose, then they turned a horrible green colour. A dentist came, looked at Ma's teeth and then pulled them all out without using painkillers. We never received a bill for her treatment.

Mother was now confined to bed with heart trouble, and she got worse and suffered from dropsy. The swelling in her tummy was enormous and about once a month the medics came to the house. They put a tap into her and attached it to a long tube and drained her stomach into a large pot under the bed. This treatment drained twenty to thirty pints and the day after the medics had been, Ma slowly got up and was moving about the house. Today, water tablets are the best reliever, but I often wonder how they can drain the fluid without removing some vitamins and minerals from the body.

Ma spent almost six years in bed with constant pain and unfortunately passed away when she was only forty-six years old. Five years on, we were still paying the doctor's bills.

About this time there were many tough characters in our area, but none like Uncle Bill Byram. He played football for a local team that later became known as Oldham Athletic Football Club. At seventeen he was over twelve stone and at thirty, well over twenty stone. He worked (as some men did) at Platt Bros., which was considered better than going to the cotton factory. He graduated into the foundary, and gained a tough job in front of the furnaces pouring boiling liquid into moulds. It toughened his body and in particular his hands.

One Saturday, after playing football, he came home to find his younger brother (Uncle Frank) lying on his favourite horsehair couch. Uncle Bill wanted to lie down as he usually did on a Saturday afternoon but Uncle Frank refused to get up. After Uncle Bill asking politely twice, he put his tough hands into the fire and pulled out a lump of coal. The coal was stuffed down Uncle Frank's open shirt and this left his chest in a right mess but he leapt off the horsehair couch. Uncle Bill dusted his hands and lay down.

CHAPTER 4

RHEUMATOID ARTHRITIS

From the age of eight, I was the only wage earner (that is after Mother could no longer work), and most of the home problems fell on my little shoulders and I started to feel pain in my legs, and my middle knuckles on each hand became sore and very swollen. By the time I was thirteen, I could hardly walk without pain; we called in the doctor and he diagnosed it as being rheumatoid arthritis and I was told to stop in bed. This was impossible, I was taking two paper rounds a day and any other job from which I could earn a few coppers. I had always fancied being a doctor and any cheap books on health, exercise and disease, I devoured. One source, was Oldham Outside Market, where I got some grubby second-hand books for only a few coppers. One book I got really inspired me, it was in a sorry state but it was all about diet, exercise, fasting and the prevention of disease. I think that this book helped me to alter my life because it taught me that health was my responsibility and that you must work at being healthy to actually be healthy. GRIT YOUR TEETH AND MOVE became my motto. Fate must have been with me when someone gave me a copy of *Health and Strength*, with my self massage, according to this book.

My difficulty in walking was helped by a chum selling me his old bicycle for two shillings and sixpence. Once I had got on the bike I managed pretty well. I am sure the exercise did me good, it was much less painful than walking and when there was a hill I walked using the bike as a crutch.

Outside our house we had some iron railings and I used to walk sideways holding onto the rails grimly.

One day our doctor caught me and he went hysterical, "You foolish lad get back into bed and rest, you are ruining yourself. If you keep trying to exercise you will be crippled for life."

Those were his exact words, I remember them very clearly.

Another doctor said to me "Mark my words Byram, you will never see twenty-one."

I am sure that I was born with a stubborn streak — still now at eighty-five the streak is still there. If somebody says that I can't do something, I will usually have a go. Brother James and I started doing exercises together, using an old iron bedstead for weight training and old bicycle inner tubes as chest expanders. James left school at fourteen and because of his still weak state, worked in a chemist shop rather than at the cotton mill.

I left school at fourteen as well but had to start at the cotton mill for twelve shillings a week. Even with my cycle and getting downhill, it was difficult getting to the mill. The hot, humid conditions seemed to suit my rheumatism and using my bike as support I could usually walk home.

Finances at home were better, and although advice was against it, I became vegetarian and kept it up for twenty years. Without a doubt, this and exercise cured my rheumatism in the next four years.

At school I had been told that my heart was not good and I was not allowed to do gym or play any sports. I loved to watch football and sometime later there was a football competition called Factory and Workshop Medal Competition. One of our workers, with a heavy job in the factory, played every night and two matches on a Saturday afternoon, as we worked on Saturday mornings. The semifinal and the final were played on the Saturday just before it got dark. This amateur centre half was Albert Pierpoint, later to be the Hangman, and a nicer lad was never born.

CHAPTER 5

STUDIES

Before I was sixteen, I had done a postal course in massage and medical electricity. I had found that I could study easily at work. In the spinning room we followed the mules, as they ran on steel lines piercing broken ends. It was an easy job but very monotonous, so I took study papers to work, fixed them on a tall can and as I walked round read a few lines. This worked well until one day the manager, who had been watching me for a while, came round and asked me what I had been reading. I told him about my studies of naturopathy. He then replied that I had no right to study anything in their time only cotton, but to my surprise I wasn't sacked. I carried on my studies in the mill and about ten years later when I had started my practice, he came to me for treatment.

Along with my vegetarianism, I started to fast; the first time being when I was only fifteen. I now know that it was dangerous to fast at that age when I was still growing but after two full days without food, the hunger had gone and I felt a lot better. The hunger and the pain had gone. I experimented with short fasts until I could eventually manage a week. I have explained more about this later in the book.

James and I joined the Westwood Health and Strength Club and started body building. James became very interested in weightlifting and despite his late start in the sport, eventually became the British 9-stone Champion at the age of forty.

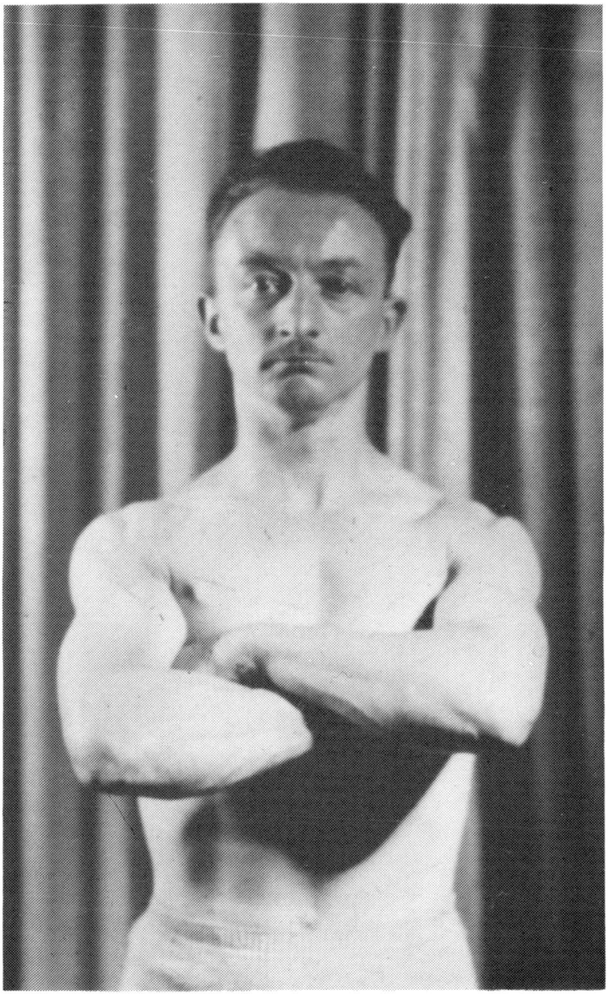

James Byram (age 40)
British 9-stone Champion

CHAPTER 6

WARWICK BROS.

My interest in massage was building strength and perhaps because my legs were weak I concentrated more on my arms. I practised hand balancing and became rather good and later joined my friend, Harry Heathcote, and we balanced together. Harry was well built with a very good posture and he became the supporter, while I was the balancer or top man. We built up a little sequence and performed in charity shows, hospitals and even in Strangeway Jail. We called ourselves the Warwick Bros.

One night in the club, a member came up to us both and said that there was a 'Go as you please' competition at the local cinema, La Scala, and first prize was ten pounds.

"What about it?" I asked him.

"I've booked you in for Monday night."

"No way!" we both said together, but after being called windy, cowards and yellow, we gave up and agreed to go to the competition. We turned up and managed a six-minute show, but we got second prize. The first artiste was a stand-up comic, who said what was then a risque rhyme — "There was a young lady called Starky, who ran off and married a darky, she paid for her sins, with three lots of twins, one white, one black and one karky."

In the next two years we won many cash prizes, which helped me to buy books and postal courses. Many amateur artistes became pros after being on these shows but for me I just carried on working in the mill and as soon as the engine stopped I dashed down the fire escape to meet Harry, who usually finished work earlier than me. A lot of

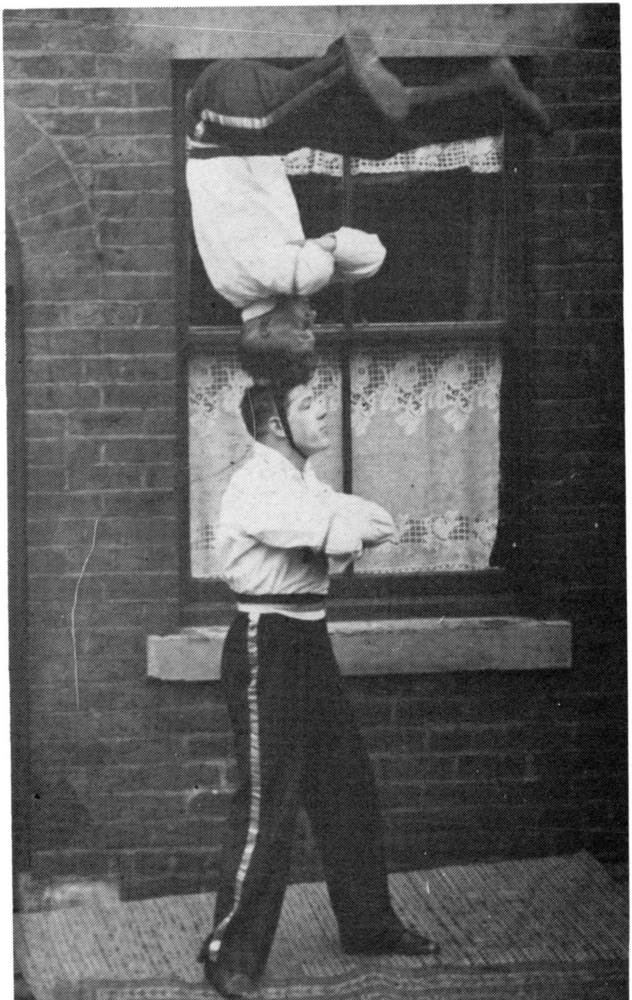

Warwick Bros. — Warwick Street (1930)

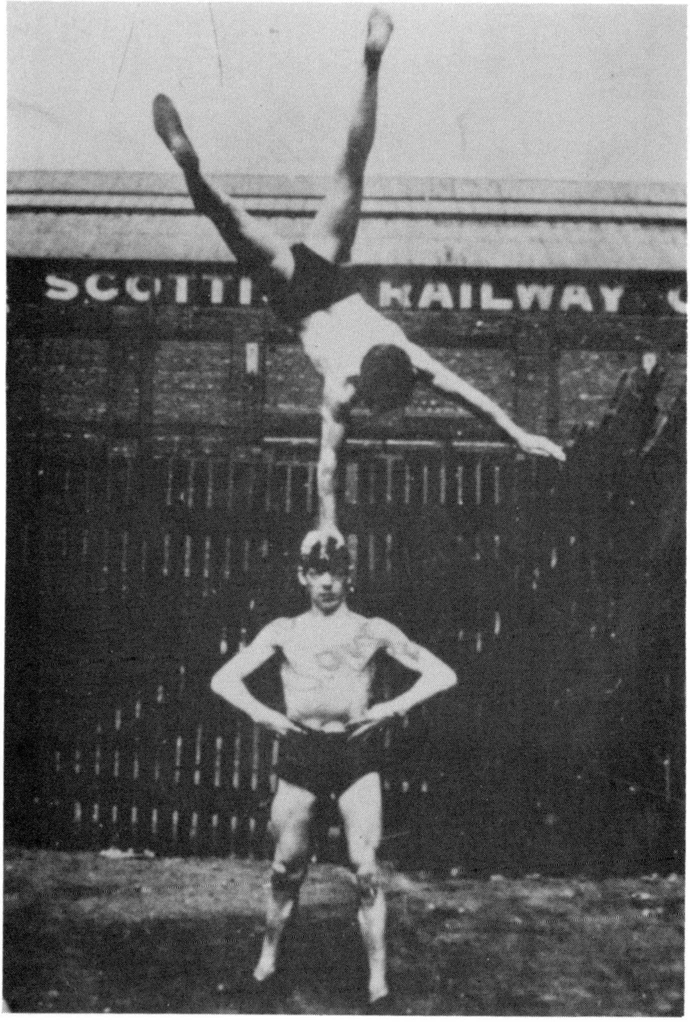

Warwick Bros. Late Teens

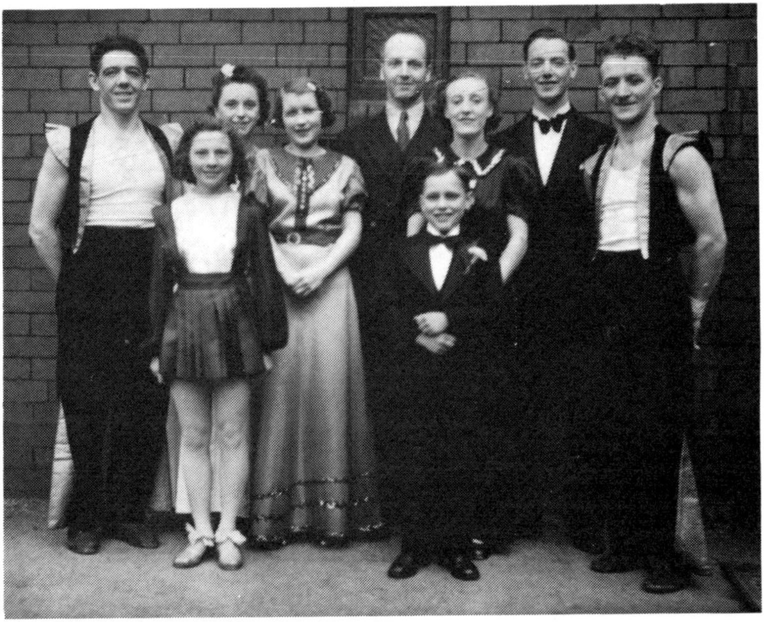

At the Gaumont — Warwick Bros. and Concert Party

the time we travelled long distances and often arrived home later than 'one' in the morning. Sometimes we would have to walk the seven miles from Manchester. I would not be allowed to slack and still was made to be at work for half-past seven in the morning.

We once won twenty pounds and a week's engagement (cabaret) at the Ritz Ballroom. The band leader was Billy Cotton. He was a real character, and adopted the call sign "WAKEY WAKEY" and his big band played worldwide. Bill's interests were flying and car racing and in his later years broke some records at Brooklands. Billy's greatest record was joining the war effort in 1914 when he was only about fifteen years old, and also seeing action abroad long before his sixteenth birthday.

We had been given offers to turn pro; one was from a great showman Syd Seymoor and his Madhatters Band.

In 1931, Syd and his band had scheduled a tour of America, but Mother was ill and I could not leave her. We were picked to appear on the London Palladium for the annual Health and Strength Show. The rail fare was then fifteen shillings return and after that first show we were asked to appear in many more displays. We were billed as the 'Ever-Famous Warwick Bros., Britain's Premier Equilibrists in Power and Perfect Balance'.

One night whilst I was in the club, I fell and displaced the cartilage in my knee and however hard I tried, I could not put it back. There was a renown bone setter in Ashton, a Mr Morley, who fixed my knee in two minutes. It was a great lesson for me. I spent every night, Saturday and Sunday at the club trying to get stronger and fitter. A few years after, I spent time visiting my early patients and started to get known.

The club had been mainly boxing but my brother and I pushed more for wrestling, gymnastics, running and weightlifting. We later banned smoking which had always lived with boxing; health became paramount.

CHAPTER 7

NAN AND PATIENTS

I had never had much time for girls, but in 1934, when I was twenty-four I fell for lovely Hannah Wright and this was another turning point in my life. We were just right for each other from the very first date. Nan, as I called her, was a victim of the cotton mill, suffering from emphysema and she also had pneumonia whilst we were courting, and many more bouts during our fifty-nine years of marriage. She was my one and only. We had no honeymoon but Harry and I did a charity show that night. In our first ten years of marriage, my Nan didn't get rid of that chronic cough. Her mother and brother both coughed, but her father who smoked thick twist tobacco, in a far from clean pipe which sent clouds of smoke round their house, never coughed once. No matter how Nan suffered, I never heard her complain or ever have a frown upon her face — she always smiled. We got married in June 1935 after buying a new sunshine house costing three hundred and ninety-five pounds. The house had three bedrooms and I used two of these for treatment once I had got established.

I continued to work in the mill, but came home and started real work at six in the evening and only finished work at about eleven at night, massaging wrestlers, rugby players and athletes. One of my early successes was a Teddy Lake who worked at the same mill as myself, but in the testing office. He suffered from severe colitis, often going to the toilet six or eight times before breakfast and sometimes he even passed blood. Teddy had been given lots of medical treatment, which didn't seem to help. As soon as he had stripped I could see that his stomach muscles were unusually tight and his posture was very bad. On questioning I had found out that he had been on crutches for eight months after he had broken his foot. It was obvious that the crutches had been too short and poor Teddy had a bad stoop and also leaned forward from the waist — thus tensing his abdominal muscles. Treatment started with infrared heat to the lower stomach area, followed by my massage to the lower chest wall and pushing the small of the back inwards, to tilt the pelvis forwards. Exercises to stretch the front muscles and plenty of back bending reduced fluid intake and I told him to spend more time chewing his food and avoiding roughage. In three months he was taller, stomach was relaxed and his colitis was cured. Teddy then said that the treatment I had given him was worth a million pounds but gave ten shillings instead.

I carried many patients upstairs and one who was a congenital spastic — Stanley Adams — was brought by his mother, two miles every Sunday morning. I had explained to her that there was no possibility of him being cured, but she told me that any help would be appreciated. We fixed a small fee between us and told her that it would never increase — it didn't — even though I ended up treating him for more than fifty years. I treated Stanley every Wednesday after I had finished working at the factory. Stanley was unable to do anything, except talk with difficulty and smile. His brain was not affected, but he still had to be fed, washed and carried. His mother worked very hard to care for him on her own, as his father had cleared off as soon as he was born, and gave him everything love could give. She was helped a lot by two wonderful people, Stanley's Uncle John and Auntie Nellie. When Stan's mother died at sixty-five, they took over and sacrificed their lives for the next thirteen years. They both died in 1990, but not before the Bishop of Salford had

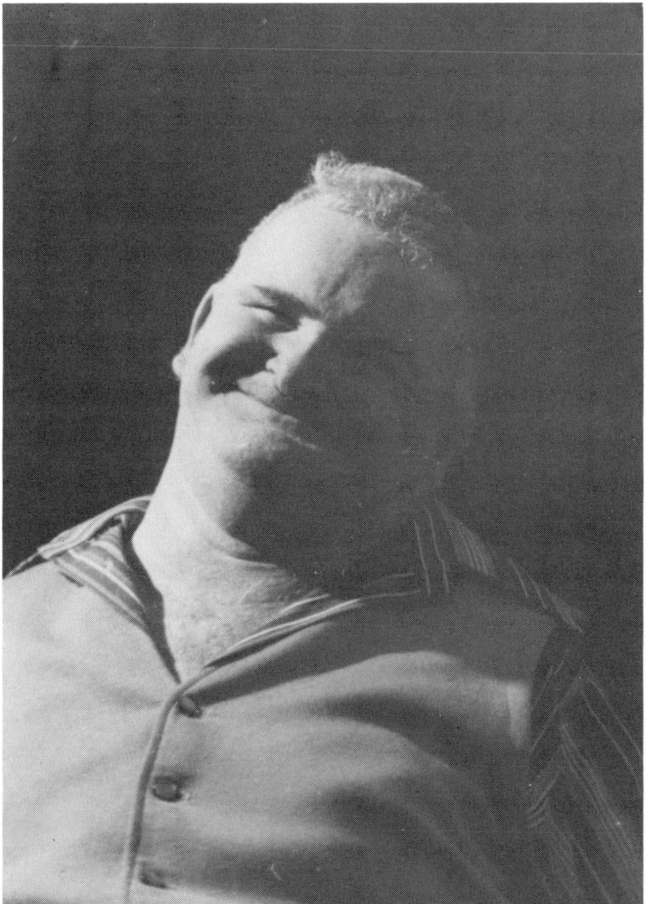

Stanley Adams

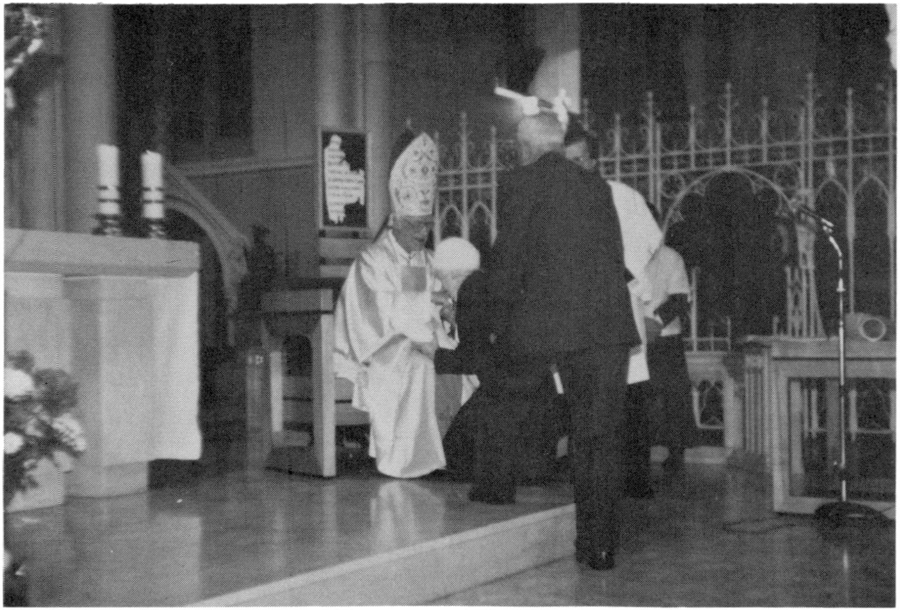

Stanley's Uncle John and Auntie Nellie receiving award from the Pope at Manchester Cathedral by the Bishop of Salford

given them medals that had been blessed by the Pope. This was the highest Catholic award for care and devotion. Stanley had then to go into a home for the disabled and old people in the area. He lived there until he passed away at the age of sixty-five.

Of the many books I read, those by Sister Kenny (the Australian nurse who successfully treated poliomyelitis) inspired me and I was eager to try her methods, allied to some of my own ideas. My first polio case was Margaret Schofield, who was two and a half years old. Little Margaret had one leg and the opposite arm paralysed. She had been given an injection in the hot summer for the diptheria virus and this had introduced the polio virus. Margaret was a tough child and made quite good progress. She eventually married, had a child, learned to drive and left Oldham to go and live near the Lake District.

Another polio patient was Wilfred Lee (aged 40) who had the unfortunate case of having both legs paralysed. Our local orthopaedic specialist gave me permission to treat Wilfred but didn't think that he would ever walk again. He could not get into a car but his cousin had a coach and brought him every lunch time. In six months he walked fifty yards, and two months later, he was back at work as a maintenance joiner at a local mill. Wilfred didn't care for inside work and later got an outside job collecting the toll fares on Shard Bridge over the River Wyre, near Blackpool. One day a car didn't stop and the poor man was badly smashed up. It wasn't long after that the poor man died.

Betty Lister was another polio victim, and again Mr Nish, the orthopaedic specialist at Oldham Hospital, not only gave me permission to treat her but also he got an ambulance to pick her up from Greenfield and drop her off at my house, twice a week. Betty's legs and arms were quite badly paralysed, but was a fighter and made great strides. Home conditions were very poor and her father had been in hospital a long time. Once we had become friendly we took her to Southport, for a Sunday trip. This delighted her, as she had never seen the sea even though she was a teenager. After twelve months' treatment, Betty was able to walk a little and so we took her to see her father in hospital, who was amazed to see her walk unaided down the ward. He cried with joy, at the sight. A few days later he sadly passed away.

I had many other disabled patients and enjoyed treating them immensely, perhaps because adversity builds character.

The greatest character on my books was David Foden, whose parents came to see me about David when he was seven years old, lying in isolation in hospital with severe polio. I told them that I could not do anything until he got out of hospital. They pleaded with me to pretend to be his uncle just to go in and have a look at him. He was paralysed from the waist down, but due to his long time left in bed, his upper body was wasting. His parents, John and Mary, pleaded for his release, but were told he must continue to rest in hospital. They came back to me, very upset, for advice on what to do.

"Go and see Mr Nish and tell him that I am prepared to give him intensive treatment when he comes out."

The next day David was released from hospital and I went to his house at ten in the evening and massaged him all over whilst he slept. I carried on doing that for almost every night for two years and he started to use crutches. He later was provided with an invalid car prior to passing his driving test. Later still he became an accountant, married a lovely lady, had two wonderful children and became the main instigator of the Oldham Owls Disabled Basketball Teams.

I could write a whole book about David, and nearly forty years on I still consider him, his parents and his wife as my top friends. My late wife loved them all. When I hear able-bodied people moaning, I think of the Oldham

Owls playing their hearts out and smiling despite pain and difficulties. Oldham Owls have played in Canada, Germany, Italy, Belgium, France and Spain and have been in the top eight in Europe for the past ten years. Currently, they are the second in Great Britain. Many of them, including David, have won gold and silver medals at Stoke Mandeville at various disabled sports and completed numerous marathons.

CHAPTER 8

NORTH WALES

After Nan and I were married, winter often caused her chest to play up, but by then I had bought infrared lamps and other apparatus, which helped. We also cut out all milk, which caused her a lot of catarrh and phlegm. Later we bought a second-hand caravan in Rhuddlan, North Wales. The air there was far better than it was in Oldham and suited Nan much better. We enjoyed this for forty-five years and again fate must have been with us, or should I say the Good Lord because I met Lord Langford. My life changed as I began salmon fishing and made some lovely new friends in this beautiful place.

On one of our weekend trips to the caravan, the site owner's brother, Sam Milligan, who knew me, asked if I could do anything for his tennis elbow. I managed to cure it with one session in the van; it was a trapped nerve in the back of his neck. The hospital had concentrated on the elbow but luckily I noticed that the radial nerve was failing in his thumb. I followed this nerve to its source in the neck vertebrae, and discovered a very painful spasm there. Soothing massage and a quick manipulation did the trick. Every weekend I got pestered by Sam, who told Lord Langford I would see him for his back troubles. I told Sam to get lost because I was here to get away from work. I eventually relented and found his Lordship very pleasant, friendly and also in quite a lot of pain. It was obviously early arthritis. This became regular treatment at Bodrhuddan Hall for the next forty years. I was treated with great kindness at all times and we eventually got known as Albert and Mrs B. On many occasions I helped some of his friends and family. It was, and still is, great to fish in his private stretch of the river. Many's the great salmon and sea trout that I luckily caught.

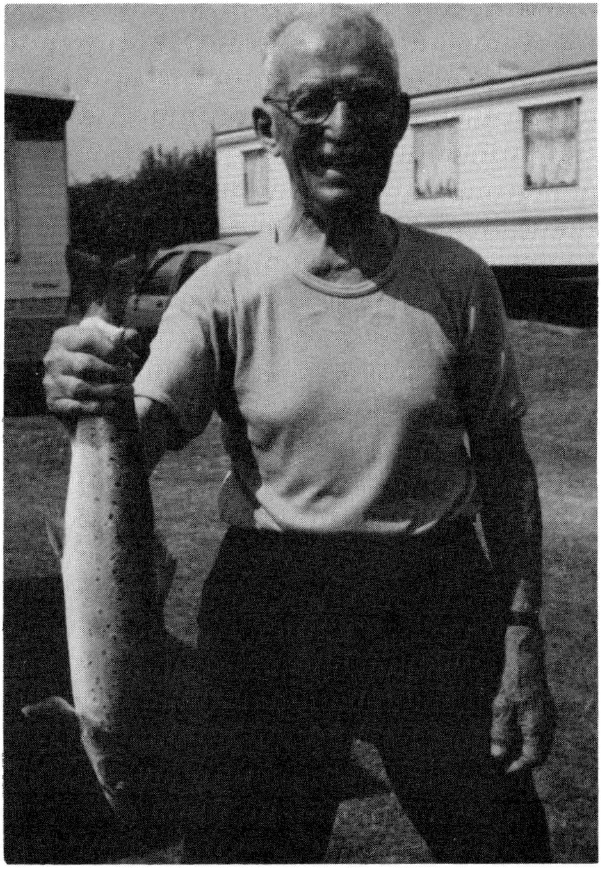

Albert's 1995 Catch

CHAPTER 9

HEALTH AND STRENGTH SHOWS

We had many keen chaps weightlifting, wrestling, running, body building and practising physical culture in all its forms. We ran health and strength shows in our small club with an audience capacity of about forty people. This brought a little money into the club because we charged sixpence for one person to get in; it also spread the health gospel and got us new members. Physical culture was booming, particularly in Yorkshire, where in the 1930s many big shows took place and the music halls were doing well, often featuring strong men. I remember once when I was there, a strong man pulling a fully-loaded double-decker bus with his teeth, all around Ashton Market. There was also a Yorkshire collier who had built up an extremely strong neck and could push coal wagons with his head, thus relieving the pit ponies. This was the man that they could not hang and at many shows, he stood smiling whilst twenty big chaps, ten on each side stood and pulled a rope around his neck to try and strangle him. They never succeeded.

I have in front of me a bill for a physical culture display, the 7th annual at a mechanics institute in Bradford. There are thirteen items on the bill, including:

R. WALKER,
Our heavyweight weightlifting champion.
THE WARWICK BROS.
A WEIGHTLIFTING CONTEST.

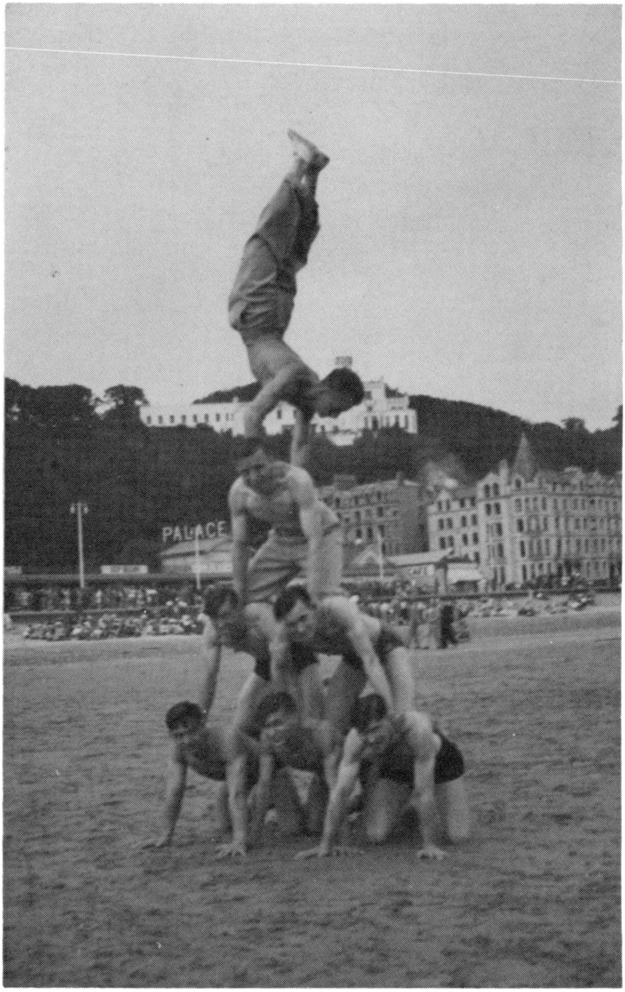

Club Boys (1934)

LADIES' PHYSICAL EXCELLENCE COMPETITION.
THE SYMETRI BROS.,
A posing act.
THE COLLEGE LADIES,
Barbell.
SWEDISH DRILL,
Acrobatic and pyramid display.
TROXY QUADS,
Strength, Grace and Balance.
OSCAR HEIDENSTAN,
1937 winner. England's best-developed man and others.
Stalls and Gallery.

One shilling including tax. All seats tip-ups and bookable.

CHAPTER 10

MANGER AND OUR SHOW

In the 1930s, Oldham had five live theatres, and in 1938 we used one of the theatres. At this time, I was the principal of Westwood Health and Strength Club and at a committee meeting it was decided that we run a big show at the Theatre Royal in Oldham. I was asked to try to get in touch with the World Heavyweight Champion Weightlifter — won at the Berlin Olympics 1936 — Joseph Manger. This was certainly going over the top — Manger lived in Freising Munich and in those days, you could only take eleven Deutschmarks out of Germany. Also the Germans had been upset that the Health and Strength cancelled (at the last hour) the proposed appearance of top German athletes at the London Palladium. I wrote first to Mr W. J. Lowry, the technical advisor to the British Weightlifting Association, and his reply, which was over eight hundred words, basically said that I would have a lot of trouble in getting him to our venture. He said that the Germans would expect the very best hotel and a companion would join him for a full week in Oldham. They would expect money first and a commemorative award. He didn't exactly say it, but it was obvious in his letter, that a few rather poor working lads would even think of holding this venture. Even the exchange rate was against us.

After many phone calls and a few letters, the Germans agreed to come to Oldham. There were many hectic preparations and now we had to fix the order of the day,

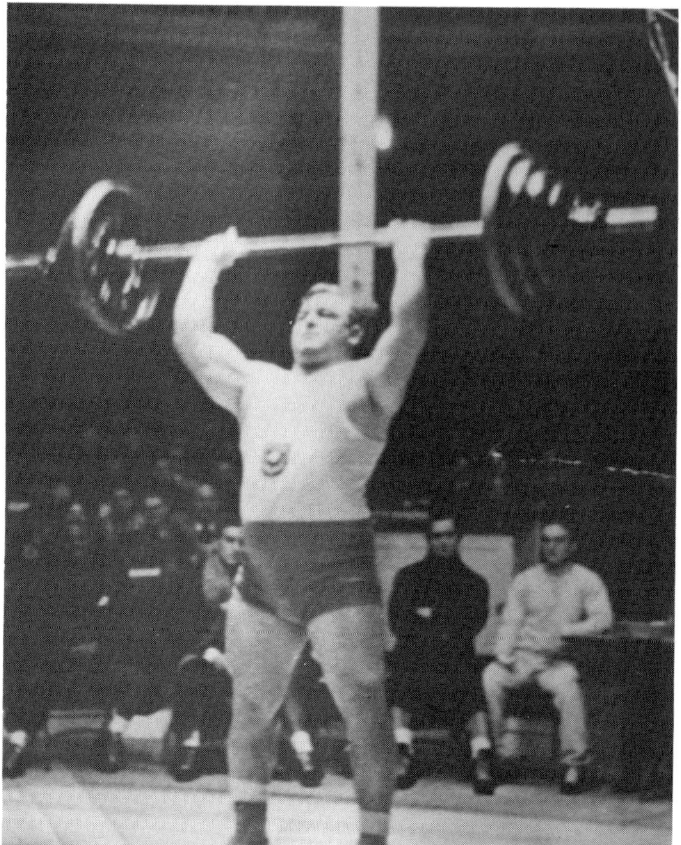

Joseph Manger — World Champion

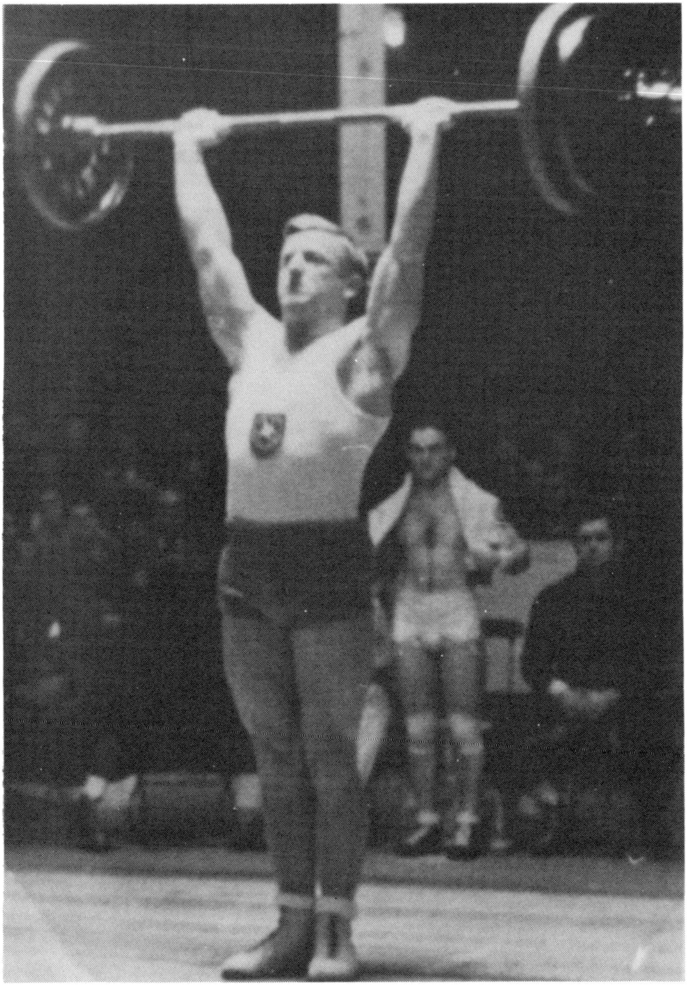

Rudi Ismayer — World Middleweight Champion

fixing programme — fixing the price of seats, and many efforts to stimulate interest.

Health and Strength helped and the Editor said that he would do what he could, and intended to be there, but the Central Council of Recreative Physical Training refused free seats. They appeared to think that weightlifting was infra dig.

But today I wonder if Germany's annexation of Austria in March 1938 and the possibility that it would be the fate of Czechoslovakia pretty soon.

One piece of good news, Manger would bring along, Rudi Ismayer, the World Middleweight Champion, who spoke perfect English — this was very welcome because none of our boys understood the German language, and I not too good at English — got in touch with all the artistes who agreed to come for bare expenses. Most advertisements were at a reduced rate, and my friend Harold Garlick printed the bills and tickets almost for free.

I met the Germans at the station and nearly passed out when they did the Nazi salute. However, I took them home, and it was evident that our small sunshine house was a surprise to them, but my wife's welcome and later her cooking — which they certainly enjoyed — soon settled them down, but we had to get a message to the milkman; Manger had ten or twelve pints each day, of full-cream milk.

It was three days before the show and every day we all went to the theatre to rehearse. The two Germans wanted to walk back from the theatre, so they bought a local map, and even though the theatre was only a mile away they must have walked for miles.

The Great Day — SAT.: 10th Dec. 1938 dawned cool and fine. I have the coloured bill in front of me now, but I would doubt if it would reproduce, so I will list the turns, especially for some of the helpers who may, hopefully still be with us.

TOP OF THE BILL
JOSEPH MANGER,
Super Human Weightlifting.
MR W. J. LOWRY,
Referee.
THE ROYAL SCHOOL OF GYMNASTS.
CARL APOLLO,
World's Strongest Man in Mighty Feats of Strength.
KENNETH and his Famous Stage Band.
MISS JOAN LAWRENCE,
Winner of England's Venus Competition.
RAMON'S and ROBINSON'S
Comedy Acrobats.
SIX SKIPPING SISTERS,
Dancing, Skipping and Acrobats.
WARWICK BROS.,
ENGLAND'S FAMOUS ACROBATS,
Pose, Poise and Power.
SENSATIONAL WRESTLING MATCH —
A FIGHT YOU WILL NEVER FORGET.

	Old Money
Orchestra Stalls	3/-
Dress Circle	2/6
Back Stalls	2/-
Unreserved Circle	1/6
Gallery	1/-

Prompt start at 2.30 p.m., but when Manger and Ismayer came on stage again I nearly had a fit — they looked marvellous — but the audience stopped cheering when they came smartly to attention and did the Nazi salute.

A few hisses and boos, but my club lads acting as stewards stopped most of it, and at once Ismayer made a speech saying there should be no politics in sports. He spoke very well and got a good clap afterwards.

On with the show which was first-class all through.

At home we had a party and as is usual we were entertained with tricks of strength or slight of hand and body.

Joseph Manger did a back somersault landing lightly despite his sixteen stone. He also easily held at arm's-length a fifty-six pound weight, but we didn't tell him that one of our club boys could write his name — Norman Greenfield — on a blackboard with a fifty-six pound ring weight hanging from his little finger.

Ismayer bent a six-inch nail at arm's-length, but we didn't tell him that a Yorkshire Strong Man could bend three six-inch nails in the same position in forty seconds. Mr Lawrence had a fifty-six pound flat weight with half a crown fixed in halfway, he gripped the outstanding half between finger and thumb, lifted it well up, put a ten-pound note under the weight and said anyone could have the note if they could do this tremendous feat. Nobody did.

Early in the evening, Rudi Ismayer asked one of the boys, Cliff Birch, to get him a few postcards of places in Oldham. Cliff managed with some difficulty and came to see me saying "What's the sudden interest in poor little Oldham?"

Late that night, the German was writing in bed for a long time — in fact I saw their light still on at 2 a.m.

They left two days later on friendly terms, and I resumed my work in the cotton mill. It was only when Oldham was bombed by the Luftwaffe, that I wondered why Oldham? Surely we didn't class as a military target? We even had German prisoners at a local mill. The nearest bomb to us was in the middle of a bowling green pub two hundred yards away. It went in deep which saved a lot of damage, but strangely a large lump of clay came through our roof. Windows were broken but no real structural damage near us, but serious damage and death in other parts of Oldham. I was away at the time but years later I still wonder.

After the show we learned something about amateur sport. When Manger showed potential before the 1936 Berlin Olympic Games, he was bought out of his small chemists' shop, given a position as Head of Tax Collecting, with nothing to do only train and enjoy regular free massage.

Our British Heavyweight — Ronald Walker — was on the dole getting eighteen shillings each week, often going to bed in the afternoon because he was hungry. Was it any wonder that Manger beat Ronald in the 1936 Games.

CHAPTER 11

HERBIE HALL AND OTHERS

One of my club chaps, Herbie Hall, became a good amateur wrestler and I suggested to him that he should try and get out of the unhealthy cotton mill. A couple of weeks later Herbie came to me to say that he had a fresh job in the moulding room at Platt's Steel Works — out of the frying pan? — but he still trained hard and eventually won the British title, and went on to win it for the next ten years — recorded in the *Guinness Book of Records.* He was picked for the Olympic Games in Helsinki, Finland, in 1952.

At the club we had a "whip-round" to help pay his expenses to London for the trials. Not a penny above the train fare was received from the Olympic Committee.

Herbie worked all day Friday, travelled to London Saturday, got kitted out Sunday and was in Finland wrestling on Monday. His opponent, an Egyptian had been in Finland getting used to the climate for six weeks. In nearly all sport Britain was the poor relation and perhaps the only amateurs. Herbie competed in the Melbourne Olympics, 1956; Vancouver Empire Games 1954; in 1958 Cardiff and in 1955 he was touring South Africa as an amateur. He started out a poor man and finished still poor. His greatest memory is being presented to the Queen and Prince Phillip at Buckingham Palace.

Sorry about this break in continuity but I still feel that we seldom treated all our athletes as they deserved.

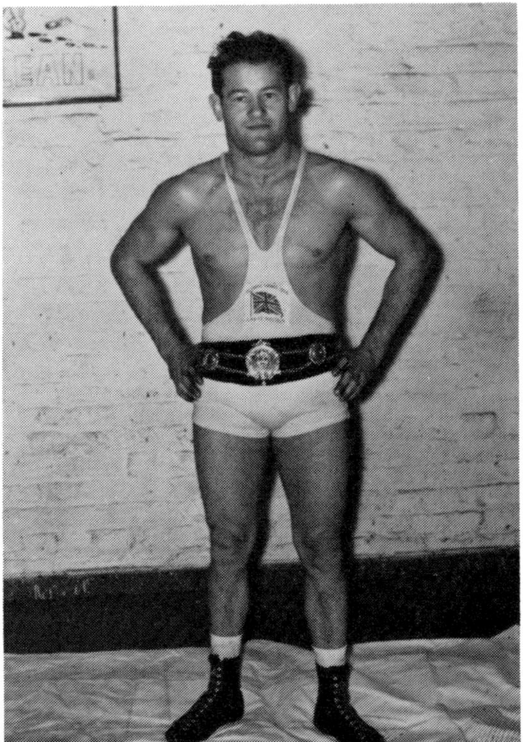

Oldham's Herbie Hall — British Champion

CHAPTER 12

BACK TO WORK AND THE CABARET

Back to work and a few more shows for Harry and I. We were booked at a top Manchester hotel for midnight cabaret, but a week prior the poor lad developed an enormous boil on his lower back; this prevented practise and it was doubtful if we could keep the booking. We had performed in hundreds of shows and never before had we cancelled.

With Harry's permission I performed a non-medical operation. In those days I used to do a treatment called cupping, which entailed fitting glass cups that had a bulb at the top or narrow end. If you think of a wine glass without a stem but instead a hole in this position and a rubber bulb fixed therc too.

In many cases of stubborn fibrositis, I warmed the glass, put it on the painful part, squeezed the bulb quite flat, and the glass stuck to the flesh, pulling some flesh into the glass by suction. These cupping glasses were bought in France, where they were often used. Ten minutes of agony and the boil burst into the glass; two days later and my chum was OK.

When we arrived at the hotel, the manager told us that the dressing rooms were closed for painting and that we had to use the back kitchen. When we switched the light on and walked in, we just looked around — there was no mirror, no seats and it was a dump. In the middle of the floor was a large copper cauldron with the next day's soup

— black soup — the black caused by hundreds of beetles swimming on the top. This was to put us off dining out for a long time. Nothing was said, we got paid, hired a taxi and went to bed at about 1.30 a.m. I had to be up at 6 a.m. for work.

At one period we worked in the theatres for Vincent Tidsley and his master singers. We did this every night for six weeks after working daily. Vincent wanted us to give up work and turn professional and he was prepared to give us the best possible start in London. I am afraid to say that he got rather nasty when we declined his offer. We both needed a rest and Mother was in bed, so there was no way that I would leave home. We were both very fit but once did a crazy two weeks doing four shows a night. We would dash off to work in a taxi, do the first show at the Gaumont in Manchester, then travel to the Osbourne Theatre in Failsworth for the second show, then back to the Gaumont for the third and then return to the theatre at Failsworth for our final performance.

One night after work, we travelled to Kendal in the Lake District to do a one-night stand — one hundred and eighty miles return — we must have been desperate or MAD. Looking back now I wonder how we managed to stay so fit with very little sleep.

There is no doubt that interest is a vital factor and once again my motto — MOVEMENT IS LIFE, STAGNATION IS DEATH was proved. My motto in the cotton mill was YOUR MAXIMUM IS YOUR MINIMUM. Today I urge people to get up and do something physical — the body does not wear out — it rusts away with too much rest.

CHAPTER 13

WAR AND THE LONG WAIT

Nineteen thirty-nine — War looked imminent and some of the club boys joined the forces. When hostilities started, I tried to join the aircrew, but I was told to go home because cotton spinning was definitely a reserved occupation.

Two years later I tried again, my work's manager told me that I was wasting my time and they wouldn't check me in. But to his and my surprise, they checked me in and said they would send my calling-up papers later.

I waited a long time for these, but finally they came and I was eventually off to Blackpool for square bashing, then to London to be kitted out. There we were placed in flats in St John's Wood.

Next morning we paraded for full injections and vaccinations. While I fully agreed with these necessary precautions, I didn't want to have any. I had never had any injections and as a very fit vegetarian, I thought that my natural resistance could cope without them. My sergeant thought otherwise, and I finished off with my cap off in front of a senior officer, who gave me a very strong lecture. Then to my surprise gave me two minutes to state my case. I explained that I was a keen student of health, a fitness freak and a long-time vegetarian. They stamped my ID in red because I had refused all injections. I was dismissed and still in the Forces.

Everything was OK in London, but each time they moved us I had the same trouble with refusing injections, and each time it got worse. I often finished up on ''Jankers'' peeling potatoes or cleaning cookhouse floors.

We went from London to Torquay to do our initial training wing and stayed there for three months. We all thought after that we would probably go abroad, but the Service didn't like to rush things and we were moved all over the country for more training:— Ten days at Scarborough, fourteen days at Aberystwyth, one week at Heaton Park in Manchester, then twelve weeks on a special course in Aberdeen, where my dear wife came to join me for two weeks. She travelled alone in jam-packed trains, mainly full of servicemen.

After all the training we went back to Heaton Park and eventually to Liverpool where we boarded the *Mauritania* for Canada. It was a horrible journey that lasted for seven days instead of the intended four. The sea was really rough and almost everyone was sick. I was in a bunk at floor level and the two above me passed everything down onto me. I don't think anyone cared if the ship went down or stayed up. We stayed fully dressed with life jackets on for the full journey. When we got to our destination, we were in trouble because none of us were smart and clean when we arrived.

CHAPTER 14

CANADA

Later we boarded the train for Moneton, Nova Scotia, Canada, the collecting centre for all the aircrews.

We settled in at Moneton, Nova Scotia, which was a transit camp. The buildings were mainly wooden and were surrounded with about six or eight inches of solid ice. The temperature was near zero degrees centigrade. To keep us busy, picks and shovels were given out and we were told to get busy on the ice.

I soon got elected onto the catering committee, as I did before in the other camps, and due to me knowing a little about nutrition, I soon complained about the food as it was worse than in Britain, where the food was being rationed.

Two days later, the catering officer was fired, after it was found out that he had thousands of dollars in the local bank.

There was a hold-up in training, so a few of us got a week's leave. A Welsh friend and I decided to hitchhike to Niagara Falls Hotel. We were picked up almost at once. The journey each way was about eight hundred miles. As soon as we got out of one car another pulled up and the driver said "Get in", he was British. We stayed one night at the Niagara Falls Hotel. It was wonderful, we had dinner, slept and then had breakfast. The generous Canadians refused to charge us.

We arrived back at camp before the week was over and there was still no sign of continuing with the training. However, three weeks later we boarded a super train for the long journey to Winnipeg, where we had bomber and gunnery training. The train was like a first-class hotel; we were treated well and the food was great. There were even clean sheets put on the bed each day, which we were not used to.

When we arrived in Winnipeg, it was a lovely clean city, but of course there wasn't much time for sightseeing. During the bombing practise someone had left the front window flap slightly open, and at ten thousand feet the freezing wind smacked me in the face before I had dropped my first bomb. I received severe frostbite to my face. I shouted for help and the pilot quickly dived, whilst I emerged covered with ice and frost. It was painful for many days.

After finishing this course, we went to Toronto for the main course in navigation. The venue was well equipped with different facilities including a gymnasium, a swimming bath and an obstacle course. I managed to do an hour every night at the gym and then finish off with a swim.

One night I was challenged by an officer. He asked me why I was in the gymnasium every night when I should have been in the barracks studying; it was a hard course and he felt I wouldn't pass it.

I told him I was very fit and therefore I did not need as much sleep as the younger lads on the course, so that while they slept, I studied. At the end of the course I was presented with a prize for being the top of the navigation course. The next day I got a commission.

There was another long wait for transport and again we were given the *Mauritania*. This time we had a good smooth voyage and sailed into Liverpool Bay. There was trouble in Liverpool Bay and we stayed on the boat for two days.

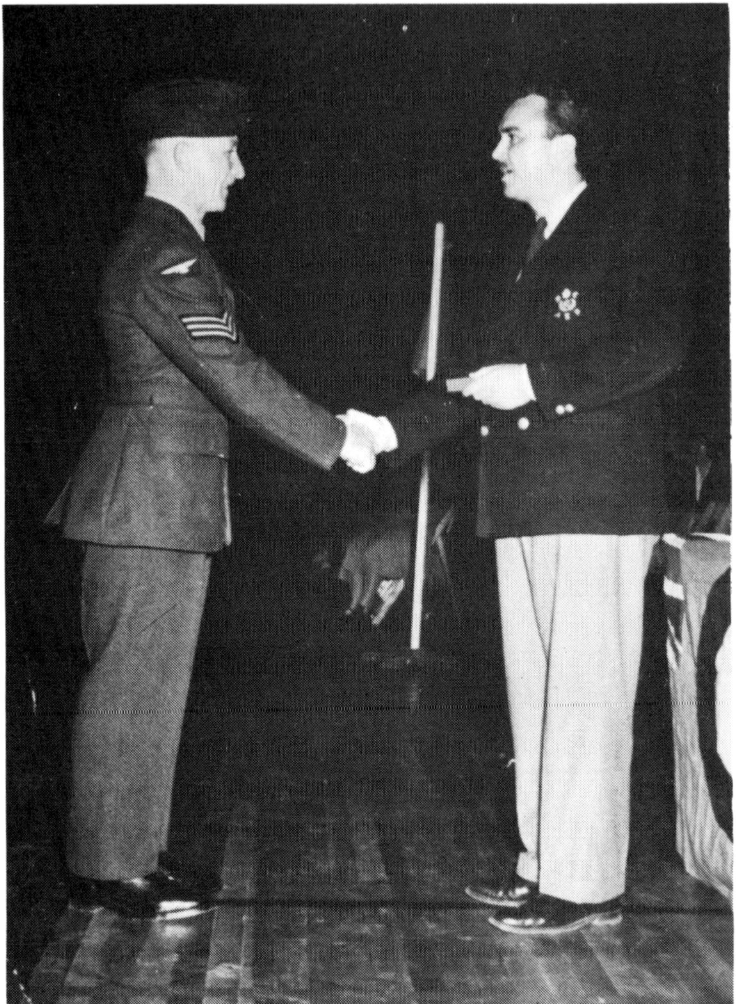

Wings Day — Canada

CHAPTER 15

HOME FOR CHRISTMAS

It was only ten days off Christmas and we were all dying to get home on leave. The next day the Customs officer boarded and asked all the officers to parade on a deck. We were asked for five pounds each, irrespective of how much we had bought back from Canada. Most of us were ladened with nylon stockings, underwear and dressing gowns etc. The Customs said that if we would pay up, they would look through our goods and they would take nothing off the other ranks.

We moved into the port, but instead of home leave we finished up in Harrogate, which felt much colder than Canada — which was zero when we left. Everyone was cheesed off until we got ten days' home leave. We received a great loving welcome. Ten days seemed to go in a flash.

We then went to Morecambe to await posting. My wife and I stayed in digs and at ten a.m. went to the headquarters to see who was on the list. After eight days I was posted. I was luckier than most and we saw those eight days together as a bonus. It was still sorrowful parting with Nan before she went home. I went to Lyneham, and some days later, I flew out to India.

CHAPTER 16

INDIA

I was put in charge of ten people. I was told that we had to stop off at about midday in Basra, in the Persian Gulf. I suggested to my men that they stuck to hot drinks, and they did not eat food with iced drinks. The temperature when we arrived at noon was about 140°F, and that was in the shade. We had all been flying at ten thousand feet at 60°F. On landing the plane, there was a mad rush to the bar where mainly sandwiches and cold beers were ordered.

Three hours later we were off again to Karachi, where we lost a few men because they were rushed to hospital diagnosed as having dysentry. I knew better — the cold drinks on top of the food had stopped their digestion and the undigested food had turned bad because of the heat — I had seen many cases of this before and saw many people with it after these cases.

At Karachi we were again in tents and we had to have injections. As usual I objected to having them. I kept saying what I believed, which was that ninety per cent of the population needed injections but that I was one that didn't. I still today think that people do not study their bodies, and therefore ignore natural health.

The next day we went sightseeing in the smelly city of Karachi. We saw a dentist sat in the kerb, with plenty of traffic on the street, taking teeth out with only a pair of nasty looking pliers. We saw a snake charmer and watched with horror as a cobra fought to death with a mongoose.

Beggars were also a familiar sight. It looked as if people had just deformed themselves on purpose to solicit rupees.

The next day whilst in the tent with ten others I heard someone shout, "Corn wallah one rupee."

By the greatest stroke of luck one chap had a very nasty corn on his big toe and I couldn't do anything about it. I offered to pay and reluctantly he agreed. The Indian had a very sharp scalpel and with fast strokes he had cut most of the corn off, almost to bleeding. Then out of a dirty pocket he pulled a little suction glass — there was no bulb with this one — but he put it over what was left of the corn and started to suck by mouth. When this was done he sealed the open end by a little gum, which was already in his mouth. He then stood up, the corn was well and truly stuck, slowly drawing out the roots of the corn, he then left it like this for two minutes. When the glass came off, the debris was inside the glass, but the toe was bleeding fairly badly. This was no problem for the man, he repeatedly hit the toe with the side of his hand and that was it. We all imagined that the toe would become infected but it healed perfectly.

There was plenty of movement around the Northern part of India before joining a squadron. I can't say that I really helped the war effort much — in fact my engagement was very little, although I saw quite a lot of India, Burma and also spent some time in Bangkok.

While near Rawalpindi, we practised dropping pack mules by parachutes; first with one chute — the poor animals broke all their four legs. Only when they were dropped with four chutes did they land softly, and even then they tended to drift from the target area.

Orders came for all personnel, including inroll followers, to proceed to Chittagong by air. I was on the last plane with the CO and staff. Unfortunately the plane in front stalled when it was just off the ground and landed in a soft paddy field. We were one kite short, but a few of the chaps in the rear seats had suffered injuries so it was back to the camp for different plans. The CO told me that I was in charge and that I must bring these people by train when they were fit to travel. So he flew off leaving me in a real fix.

After three days, I decided we could move, but what a performance at the railway station. This was mainly because I wanted a private carriage, and a wagon to put some Sten guns and ammunition; which had been left from the crashed plane. It took two days of arguments and threats to get permission. But suddenly a signal from Calcutta moved the opposition and we were off on a journey of about two thousand miles on rough uncomfortable trains. The winds were very hot and the temperature was in the nineties. We were not looking forward to this long trip. I posted two chaps with the arms and ammo; but as the days got hotter they complained of heatstroke so I got two padlocks off my baggage and locked the big door and put the sentries in with us.

After three days and three nights, we arrived at Calcutta, where we had to change onto a narrow gauge line, but when I went to the back of the train to the covered wagon, the contents and the wagon were missing. My face was red and I couldn't stop shivering despite the temperature. I could visualize myself in jail or even being shot.

After getting no help at Calcutta Railway Station, I decided to give the boys two days' leave. There were loud cheers all around. Taking a sergeant we travelled back up the line, with little optimism. Fifty miles back we found our wagon shunted in a siding with my locks still on it. Getting back to Calcutta took sixteen hours. There were no more incidents from Calcutta to Chittagong. I reported to the CO after asking everyone if they would back me up in saying that the train kept breaking down — as they often do in India. My knees were knocking and I was in a "blue funk", but the CO accepted everything. He told me to go to the "mess" to get a good meal because I looked shocking. I couldn't eat much, but as I left the Officers' Mess, a little Indian stopped me and said, "You good officer, Sahib me, tell your fortune, only one rupee."

I told him to get lost. "You can't tell fortunes, if you can, tell me how old I am."

"Sahib write it down first."

Then I did making sure that he could not see, but I wrote 53.

"Put it in my hands," said the Indian — he looked at me in the eyes and said, "Sahib joking, Sahib 35 not 53."

I gave him the rupee, and was amazed for about ten minutes when he told me uncanny knowledge about myself. Most of the things he told me came true much later on in life. The very first thing he told me was never ride on horses. This was very strange, as three weeks before I had been thrown off a rather sprightly horse, and was still in some pain. This happened two thousand miles away from him and none of the camp knew anything about it, so there was no way he could have known what had happened.

As I have got older, I have realised what stupid sense there is in the glory of war, and I abhor the films, books and plays that try to show the glorifying experience of killing humans. I would now like to recall the happier times that I saw in the war.

At Chittagong, I met a Flight Lieutenant, DFC and Bar, called Ground at 1100 hours on Thursday. The CO evidently had not noticed this and there was a good turnout on Thursday morning. HP got dressed up in his best suit and had even found a fireman's helmet. He lay a long fuse and put the medicine ball in the barrel, then stood a long way off "Short Tom". Nothing happened until a Lancastrian voice shouted "It's a bloody dud," and with that Short Tom let out a mighty bang, which blew out the back of Short Tom, but the medicine ball soared over the field and away through some trees. The next sight was a lot of Indians shouting and running in all directions. There was no damage, just a lot of dirt and dust in the nearest huts. The firing of Short Tom got me confined to camp for ten days.

After joining my unit at a small village called Guhatti, I was very interested in the Leper Hostel, and I received an invite, which to me was most interesting. When I arrived at the hostel, outside was a man lying in the sun on a prayer mat. The poor leper's legs and arms were rotting away, yet he smiled at me as I entered the building. I spent a couple of hours inside the hostel but, unfortunately as I was stepping out a few of our officers were walking past and saw me. When I got back to the mess, they all walked away from me. The word had got round that Mad Byram had been in The Leper Colony.

We had been skipping all around Bangkok and later Singapore, with a sinking feeling in my stomach that I should be at home with my wife, as word had got to me that she was ill. Instead of being at home, the powers that be sent me a signal to proceed at once to Hong Kong. I ignored this message because I was six weeks overdue for demob and wanted to go home.

A week later, a signal from Air Headquarters India for F/O Byram to proceed on release forthwith to Bombay and request air passage to UK. It was signed by the Air Commodore at Headquarters in Malaya.

We arrived in Bombay, after a few thousand miles on a train, and as soon as we arrived we met trouble; there was a smallpox epidemic. The Medical Officer, who was just one rank higher than myself, got rather nasty when he saw my no injections on my form. He told me that I was having the injection, and talked about getting help to force me into it. I ended up not having the injection and spending seventeen days in solitary confinement. I have still got a chit with his name on it, which he called Strict Quarantine.

CHAPTER 17

HOME TO A FOUR-BEDROOMED BUNGALOW

After this I flew back to Great Britain and got my demob at Wednesford and left for home the next day. I felt very guilty when I saw my poor dear wife. As most of us know the people at home often suffered more than the people abroad.

My wife and I immediately took a holiday in the Isle of Wight and I started work for a few weeks in the cotton mill, as well as picking up on old and new patients.

I had finished in the mill by Christmas, by which time I had got enough patients to fill most hours of every day. We were at the time looking for bigger premises, and in 1949, got a four-bedroomed detached bungalow which had been built by an old patient of mine in 1930. The phone seldom stopped ringing in the new house and Nan attended to this, and also settled worried children and nervous ladies with her tact and sympathy.

For years I treated many people, including lots of celebrities, police chiefs, MPs and most of the local mayors and mayoresses. Distance didn't stop people from coming; I have had many come from Scotland, Wales, South of England and a few from London. One businessman came regularly in his Rolls-Royce early in the morning and wanted to be back at his business in London at eleven in the morning. Another patient, Joseph Zaronaf, the top all-in wrestler, came from London, in a noisy four-litre Ferrari which wakened up the neighbours.

I have many testimonials which I can now look at and feel I did fair work which I always enjoyed. I would now like you to read one dated 10/07/86.

Dear Mr Byram,

I would like to thank you very much for seeing my wife on Tuesday last, and bringing her much needed relief from pain in her neck. She had been suffering great pain for some weeks and had been unable to sleep on account of it. Now she is sleeping normally and the pain has abated.

The first time my wife came to see you was when she was only twenty-three and as a recently-trained nurse, had sustained an injury to her back, while carrying out her nursing duties, and at the time, medical advice was to give up nursing; but your treatment was immediately effective and in fact she kept on working for another thirty years prior to retirement during the last Health Service reorganisation.

From time to time she had to call on you for help, and on every occasion you treated her with great kindness and understanding, and what's more, effectively. I feel bound to say that you could not have grown rich on the modest fees that you charged, and I can only hope that you will receive due reward in another place.

Over the years we have referred many of our friends to you and also members of our family who have been in trouble. All of them afterwards have sung your praises, and you may remember my wife's sister who travelled from Southern Ireland on more than one occasion to receive treatment at your hands.

Long may you continue with your good work,

Kind Regards,
H. W. Sellers.

CHAPTER 18

EXERCISE

It is not possible to be healthy unless one does some form of exercise. The body deprived of movement slowly stagnates, the circulation slows down, the organs and muscles lose tone, elimination becomes difficult, and often the mind and willpower weakens.

It isn't necessary to do a lot of things to keep your body in working order. I am not thinking of body building, weightlifting, athletics and famous sports people. The average person doesn't want to break records, doesn't want to go to the gym, doesn't want to do a marathon; just usually wants to be a little fitter without straining, panting, groaning or sweating.

All you need to do are my bed exercises, walk two miles daily, have a sensible diet, including fresh fruits and salads; but please, don't overeat — always leave the table still hungry.

Lower back pain is forever on the increase and is probably more common than the common cold, or more common than the rapidly growing asthma. Back pain sufferers increase yearly and very little appears to be done to relieve it, or to find out the real cause.

Is back pain caused by less and less movement? Muscles that are not used, tend to waste away — Use 'em or lose 'em! The modern man certainly doesn't stand on his two feet enough to prevent back pain. He doesn't walk enough, their excuse is that they have a hard working job, but most ladies stand and walk more than the average male —

housework, shopping, cooking and washing, whilst their husband sits down and watches the television or reads the newspaper. The result of this is that most ladies are healthier, have less strokes, less heart troubles and even less cancer.

MOVEMENT IS LIFE!

I knew a youngish man whose motto was don't stand if you can sit — don't sit if you can lie. He sadly passed away in his early fifties. Don't let your muscles go to pot, muscles that are hardly used degenerate fast, breathing gets more shallow and your bowels slow down. The quality of life goes with inactivity and walking and standing gets progressively harder. It is said that the primitive man could stand for hours with ease. The way to improve, is first to stand more often; the second is to learn to use muscle tone and relaxation.

In the lower back muscles, some called erecta spina (which is what they should do — erect the spine), we have lost a vital something. The following exercises will prove that we have lost it.

When many people stand upright on their feet for fifteen minutes they faint. We must try to improve our standing time by standing more often.

Along with other chemical elements, calcium is the main builder of tough bones and by standing and putting all the body weight on our legs, we are drawing calcium into the lower bones, but, this only happens when we exercise or stand, and at this point the calcium is fully attracted to the bones used. Bones without calcium get soft and spongy and eventually we can develop osteoporosis. If the calcium is left in the bloodstream, it is possible that it could be hardening the blood vessels and causing arteriosclerosis (hardening of the arteries).

However, I do know, that when we both stand and walk, we are strengthening the muscles and the bones in our body. Any exercise improves tone and strength at first, but if you keep doing exactly the same, the gain stops. You must gradually increase the effort or do more repetitions to keep improving. You may say that at first the pain is worse — true, but you are using muscles that at first may have been dormant, but as your posture gets better, your pain will be less. There is a subconscious electrical stimulus in the postural muscles, these are almost lost in the present-day man.

As we stand much more, this response can return in allowing us to stand much easier.

This hardly-understood action, allows certain fibres of the postural muscles to rest in turn, while others take the strain, maintaining enough tone to keep us erect. This act can only come when we stand a lot; so try to stand while you are using the phone, or any other task you usually sit down to do. You don't need to stand to attention, with your chest out, shoulders back, chin up and stiff back making all your body weight go onto your heels. Stand easy, with your weight slightly on your toes, let your arms hang loosely at your sides with your knees just pressed back to lock them. This way we can have bone to bone at the knee joint, relieving muscle.

You don't have to do vigorous exercise; forget touching your toes or bending your back. Exercise is to regain posture and to get control of your postural muscles.

Please spare three minutes in bed each morning for your daily exercise:—

Under the bedclothes, lie face up, first press your head back into the pillow — hold for a count of three then relax.

Sink your whole body into the bed for a few seconds — try to think of nothing and do this after every exercise.

Now, roll your head to each side. Relax.

Lift the forearms, grip your fists, press elbows into

the bed — hold for three, then relax.

Now press upper back hard into the bed — count to three, then relax.

Now press your middle back into the bed and count to three, then relax.

Now press the lower back into the bed — count to three, relax. While still pressing down, push lower part of back to the left — count to three, now press the lower back to the right — count to three, then relax.

Tighten your buttocks. Tighten your stomach muscles, and raise left leg about twelve inches forcing against the bedclothes — count to three, then relax. Repeat this exercise with the right leg. Always keep the leg straight and stiff. Repeat this exercise, lifting both legs together. Note how the stomach muscles contract when you lift both legs together. Count to three, then relax.

You are now aware of relaxation and contraction in muscles.

Now with both legs stiff, press the whole leg into the bed. After the count of three, relax.

Next, bend the knees a little, press the heels down into the bed and slide them up towards your buttocks — about twelve inches is enough, then relax.

The last exercise is to keep your legs straight and bend your ankles as far up as possible. This stretches your calf muscles. To relax wriggle your toes.

By now you have gained co-ordination of the lower muscles and every week you should increase the length of contraction in the muscles by one second.

Those are the morning exercises. Breathing is very important while exercising, so after doing all the exercises, take three or four deep breaths — in through the nose and out through your mouth — still supine.

You are now doing something to help yourself.
More movement means less pain.

CHAPTER 19

MARRIED — GOLDEN WEDDING AND THE BURGLAR

Nan and I were both twenty-five when we married, and in 1985, when we were both seventy-five, celebrated our Golden Wedding.

The Oldham Evening Chronicle came to the house to take some photographs of us. Although it was windy, he wanted me to do a handstand on the chimney. It was rather difficult because the photographer kept shouting "Hold it", whilst he walked around the street shooting from different angles. I was just about to collapse when he took the last snap. This was a salute to my grand wife.

A few years later we had a burglar very early in the morning. He was twenty-five and had got into our house by smashing a double-glazed window. He had actually got in without me hearing him. After disturbing the downstairs treatment room by throwing X-ray plates and other important things all over the room, he went into the kitchen and knocked over the microwave; perhaps he didn't think anyone lived above because he had switched on the light. I told Nan not to move because we had a burglar downstairs, but as fast as I got out of bed and went downstairs, Nan was behind me despite her poor condition. We eventually got the man on a chair facing the front door. Nan stood over him while I telephoned the police, put all the lights on and unbolted and unlocked the heavy door. In less than ten minutes five policemen and

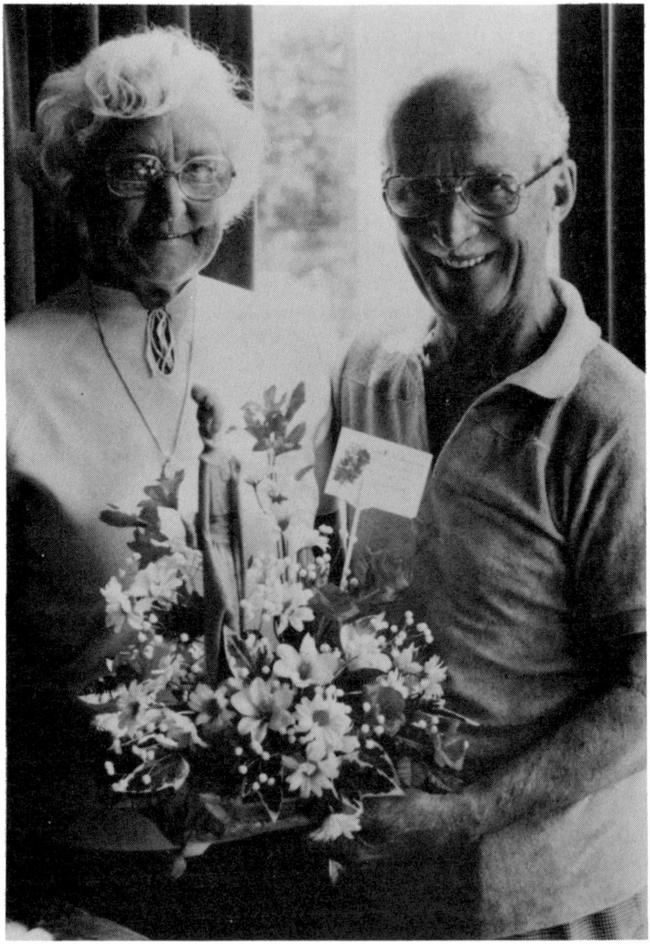

Golden Wedding Day
(Photo provided by *Oldham Chronicle*)

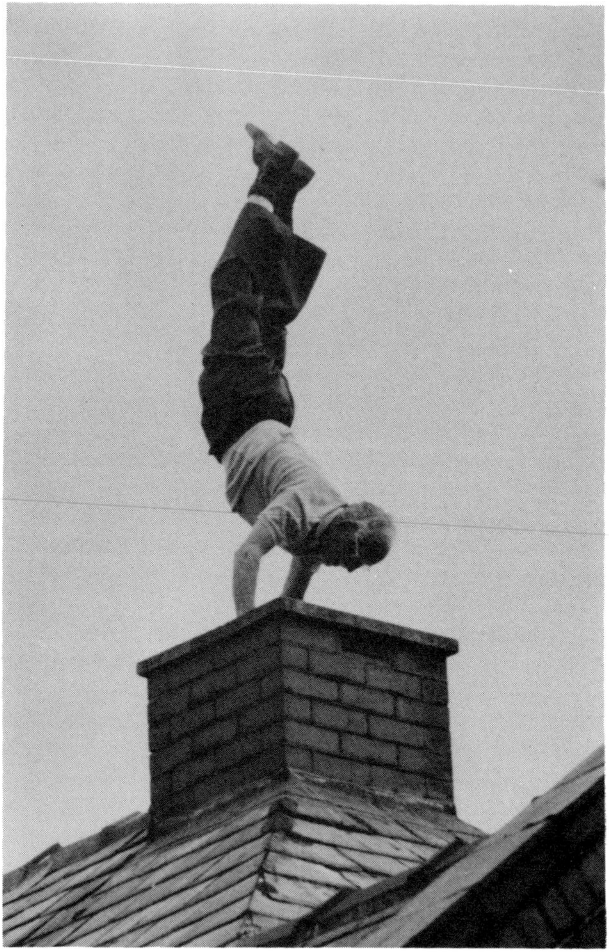

High Jinks on the Golden Wedding Day

one policewoman arrived; they carted the man off to hospital to attend to his wounds.

He later got six months in jail.

That morning my wife was wonderful but, for months afterwards she couldn't sleep — any little noise and she was up looking to see what it was. We had a story published in *The Oldham Evening Chronicle* with the headlines: "Two Old Age Pensioners Capture Burglar at 4 a.m. in Everton Road". There are only four houses in the road, so most people knew it was us. I don't know if this encouraged burglars or not.

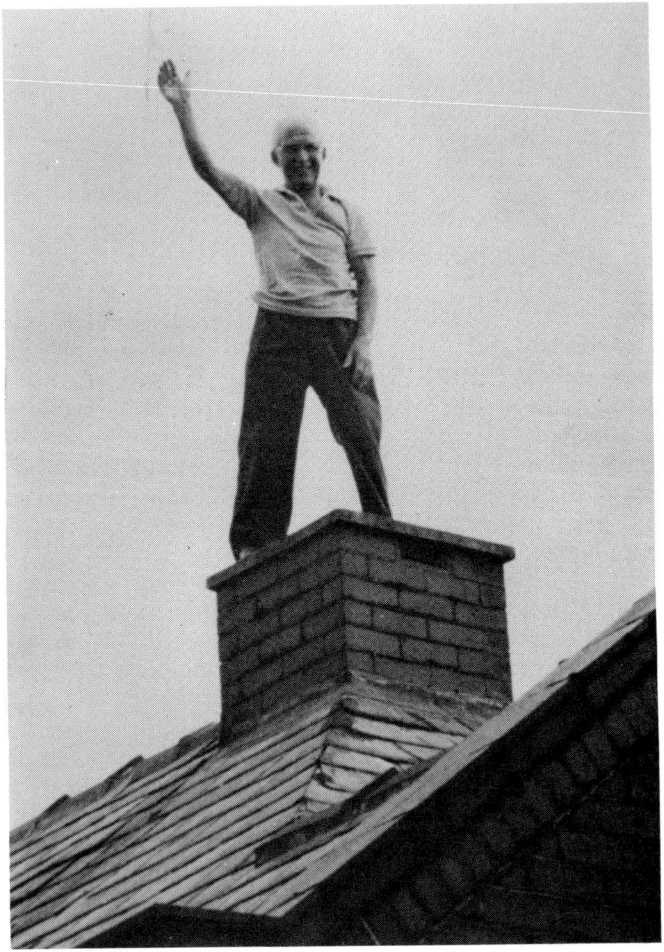

Salute to Nan on our Golden Wedding Day

CHAPTER 20

HERNIA

Shortly afterwards I had a patient whose sacroiliac joint was twisted and he was in great pain. He was nineteen stone and six foot two inches tall, and I had difficulty in getting him to relax. I pressed on regardless and using all my strength managed to snap his sacroiliac joint in.

I heard the snap and at the same time I heard my groin rip, at the same time I felt it go as well, I thought it was an inguinal hernia. The man got up and walked out alright, but I had to lie down.

My injury required an operation but I could not go and leave Nan alone in her condition. With a strong rupture belt, I managed to carry on working for six painful months. Then, once again Nan's chest caused anxiety and she was rushed into hospital.

After seeing my very good doctor, I made an appointment to go to hospital and have my hernia seen to. I rang the surgeon and was in for the operation the following Sunday. I started to fast when I heard about the operation, and when I got down to theatre it had been four days since I had eaten anything; I had just drunk water.

After the operation, I slept for ten hours; I felt fine and had a shower after I had woke up. I think someone told sister because I got a tongue-lashing off her; this was because I told her I had been fasting for nearly five days and I needed water. She pointed out the notice above my head, it read "nil by mouth", but I knew that I was dehydrating, so as soon as she was out of sight, I jumped out of bed and drank two pints of water from the patient next to me, he didn't realise — he was fast asleep. I started to eat a little, felt great and had a smashing rest. I was ready to go home, but was told that they would keep me in until Nan was ready to go home with me. Unfortunately we never had any children, so there was nobody at home who would continuously care for me.

Three days later I got word to get dressed because Nan and I were going home, but much later in the afternoon the trip home was cancelled as Nan was declared not well enough to travel, so I went home alone.

It was a bad day and it was snowing and cold, but the heating had been on all the time we were in hospital, so the house was warm. I crept into bed as soon as I got home and slept until dawn, when I fell out of bed vomiting with an incredibly bad headache. I crawled to the phone and rang for help and unlocked and opened the front door. This act probably saved my life. I had gone to bed without opening the windows and had a very bad dose of carbon monoxide.

The environmental people came and sprayed everything in the house and opened all the windows. One of them stayed with me a couple of hours. It was very close and if Nan had been home with me she would not have survived. (There is more about this later.)

We once knew a girl who lived in Portugal and she had died from carbon monoxide poisoning.

Nan and I were in a fairly large villa, but opposite were flats, three-storeys high. They had one chimney between the three flats and a gas heater in each room. The two English girls, that we had become friendly with, had had a bath each, using the gas heater and then gone to bed. One woke up in the middle of the night with carbon monoxide poisoning; she was very ill. The other girl sadly did not wake up.

There was a panic and extractors were put in every flat.

CHAPTER 21

MOTORING IN YUGOSLAVIA

As my wife got somewhat better, I resumed my driving, passed my test in my prewar Standard Flying Ten, and started thinking and planning motoring holidays abroad.

On the first holiday we flew with the car just over the Channel because I wanted to know if my dear wife's chest would cope with the changes in altitude when we flew. The journey was only about thirty miles but she really enjoyed it and felt fine all the way through the flight. This was good. Now we could fly to Australia. When we did so, she was fine.

In 1951, along with two good friends, we put our new white Ford Zodiac on the train at Ostend, and boarded the comfortable sleeper train to Milan. Once we got there we travelled by car into Venice, and stayed there for one night.

The following day we rode down to Yugoslavia. We were stopped at Customs and quickly separated. The car was checked thoroughly. It was as if we were a danger to the Tito's Empire. From then on they appeared to keep track of us as long as we were in their Empire. They knew where we were and on returning they knew exactly how much money we had spent. The journey was incredible, but it was such a beautiful country, especially inland.

There were no tourists in those days, and petrol pumps were often two hundred miles apart. One night we had to knock hard on a garage door to get petrol. It was a surprise

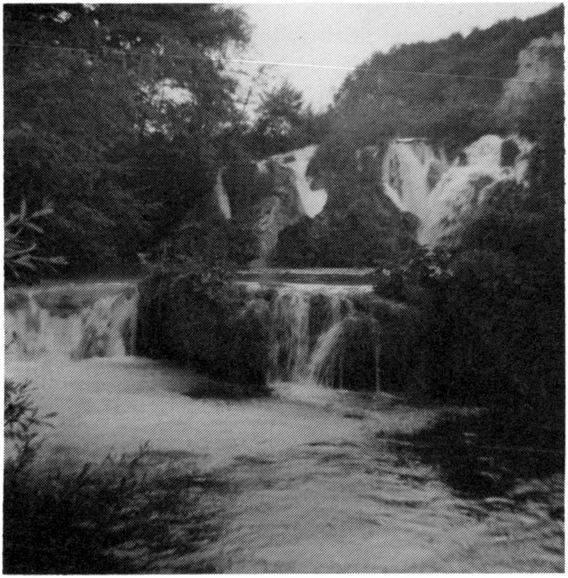

Plitwice Lakes and Falls, Yugoslavia

when he opened the door as he levelled a shotgun at us. After the panic, we offered him half a pound of English butter. He took it gratefully and started to fill up the tank from small barrels, using the world's largest tun dish which we had to hold.

When we arrived in Split, in Yugoslavia, we were most surprised to see the Bell View Hotel still open. We booked in for two days. I was carrying the cases up to our bedroom, which was very nice, and as I came down to pick up the final case there was a six-foot man, probably about twenty stone, leaning against the car demanding a parking fee. This was about two in the morning and there were no other cars around. He looked pretty mean and carried a badge of identity, so he must have only been doing his job. I paid him; the fee was about two shillings.

It was a very nice rest, with good food and excellent swimming facilities a short distance away.

Whilst still motoring south, I took a corner a trifle fast and caused a bit of tyre squeal. There was no traffic about so I was causing no obstruction, but two minutes later a large motorcycle pulled up in front of us and caused me to slam the breaks on very hard. The policeman strolled up to the car and said something to the effect of "GET OUT". Naturally we obeyed his orders, he indicated that we were to be fined. I objected to this, but he reached for his revolver attached to his belt and I immediately gave in and paid the fine. The fine was equal to seven shillings.

On our way back, we went inland to visit the sixteen lakes with the beautiful waterfalls. This was paradise and it is pathetic to think of what humans are doing to this wonderful Earth of ours.

CHAPTER 22

INTRODUCTION TO THE ALGARVE

Next fate began, when after the war, we bought a four-bedroomed bungalow, enabling me to give treatment on the ground floor. I phoned a young chap — Arnold Taylor — who repaired medical apparatus in London, asking for a large infrared lamp. At lunch time, an open sports car arrived with this eight-foot lamp hanging out of the back. My wife said to me as he was leaving "That lad will go places" and indeed he did. About ten years later, the Arnold Taylor organisation was selling in Europe, South Africa and Canada. Three years after I had received this quick delivery, Mr Taylor sent me a letter to say that he was opening a Health Centre in the Algarve, Portugal and had engaged a very good masseuse. I thought here goes fate again and at once booked, taking my wife and an elderly patient, Mrs Lewis, who would get treatment and a holiday. The cost, including a detached villa, flight from Gatwick and dinner in a lovely thatched restaurant, which by local law was obliged to serve free, a carafe of local red or white wine, was sixty-five pounds for two weeks. This was the start of many holidays in healthy Algarve. Quite a few of these holidays were enjoyed with David's parents John and Mary Foden.

After this we spent a lot of great holidays in Portugal's Algarve. The first time we travelled by car down through France and Spain, but in 1965 an airport was built in Faro, and from then on we went by plane and booked a car for the two weeks that we stayed there. We were there in the Revolution in 1974 and we were held up at the airport by armed soldiers on the way home. It looked doubtful that we would ever get home. David's parents were with us and we decided to get out table and chairs and started to play our favourite game, whist. Some of the Revolutioners came to see us and watched us play; they then joined in and found the game very enjoyable and very difficult. Although hours passed while we played the game, the condition in Spain was still bad and we were sent back to the villa. The panic was over the next day and we got a plane home to England.

During the three short trips to the Algarve, we had three small bumps in the hired car. First a big car backed into us, for no apparent reason, and they pushed the radiator in. The man refused to tell me his name and address, but seeing as though he was bigger than me, I decided not to argue with him. Once back in the car I took his registration number and rang the car hire garage. The owner of the garage was a British man who had started business with ten Minis — his name was Keith Vaughn. The business was built by good service in to a thousand car effort, but sadly he got killed by an army vehicle before he reached his fortieth birthday.

When I explained to Keith who had hit us, he did not seem that bothered. I asked him why and he replied "That's OK, he is the local millionaire, he will probably buy me a new car to replace it."

I couldn't believe it that when we went back again and hired another car from Keith, the same millionaire bumped into us again. This time he was coming out of a side street and bumped into the side panel of our car. It didn't appear to bother the millionaire and the case never went to the police.

CHAPTER 23

NAN'S MOTHER

In between holidays, I was fully occupied with many patients and when my father-in-law died, we fixed up Nan's mother in the small bedroom. She lived with us for twelve years, suffering from paralysis agitans; we gave her Arrtain tablets and kept the shaking to a minimum.

Nan's mother was able and could go out but one day she fell and broke her leg (neck of the femur). At this point she was eighty years old and had never been in hospital before. It was a great shock to everyone, especially Ma, being forced to stay in bed with one leg strung up in the air. After one month we brought her home. Mr Nish told us before we left that they were unable to operate with her being so old, so the joint would be very weak and if she did live through this ordeal then she would never walk again because of it being a very weak joint. However, six months later Ma walked with the aid of a stick down Rhyl's Promenade.

Ma lived till she was eighty-six and the fall was a great shock to her. From the time of the fall, till when she sadly died, she never shook and never took another pill. Ma loved salmon and sea trout and she expected me to catch a fish every time I went fishing, which was very often, as it was a great hobby of mine.

On her eighty-second birthday, the house was full of flowers. One of the Nolan Sisters came for treatment on her bad back; the others came to support her. After the treatment these lovely talented girls went into the lounge where Ma was sat and entertained her for about half an hour. After this she never stopped talking about the lovely girls, and when they were on television, Ma would sit totally involved.

At eleven one night, the door bell rang and an old patient, Basil Goldstone was stood at the door with a gorgeous girl who had displaced her coccyx by falling on the ice. She was the French star of the Chu Chin Chow Shoe at the Palace Theatre in Manchester. When I asked her why she hadn't gone to hospital, she told me that when she had done the same in France, she had the coccyx (tail bone) put back by a local bone setter. She asked me about my experience in this area and I told her that I had done it before. I didn't tell her that I had only done it once.

After infrared to the damaged coccyx, I managed to manipulate the bone externally. To do this I used the back edge of a small book and the muscle pad below my right thumb. The fall on the ice happened only that night, so the joint had not had time to settle in the new wrong position and no real spasm in the muscles was evident. The manipulation was successful and she appeared in the next show.

A week later we got an invitation to afternoon tea in the main dressing room with all the stars of the show and got free tickets to have the best seats in the house. It was for a Wednesday which was great, as Wednesdays were my half days. It was great entertainment even in the dressing room.

The sequel to this was being offered to be the theatre's physio. I had to refuse this offer because I already had more work than I could really handle.

CHAPTER 24

DRIVING

My work was certainly time-consuming, and I still kept my interest when some driving enthusiasts came close to me teaching advanced driving. This was called the League of Safe Drivers. I joined in 1975 and started going to the Sunday morning lessons and by 1976 had passed my Gold Award. Three years later they took their classes away from Oldham but I found myself another wonderful group near the centre of Oldham. It was called the Institute of Advanced Motorists.

I trained with the men and women who were as dedicated as me and passed the Advanced level as well as doing the skidpan exercise. I passed again when I was eighty-five. If only more people could follow these dedicated motorists we could cut down the terrible loss of lives on our roads. So many of these accidents are avoidable but so often the blame is put on anything other than the motorist. Everyone could get more pleasure out of their cars by training. You learn how to take care of it and how to be in more control, so the vehicle will last longer and passengers will feel safer. Their motto is CAR SAFETY AND PASSENGER COMFORT.

It would be great if many of the young drivers had a go at the Advanced level. I can ensure them that the instructors are able and ready to pass anyone on the knowledge and the skill that they have already.

One of our most enjoyable motor trips abroad was when we took a semi-disabled patient with us and dropped her in Rheinfelden, Switzerland, before driving through Italy and France before picking her up at Calais.

This trip was made about forty years ago, and the lady who had a back injury, and lost her husband suddenly, had taken in a boarder at the house to supplement her income.

At the time she had a man from Rheinfelden, Switzerland, who had come to a large bakery near Oldham to teach them continental icing and new methods of baking in different ways. Joseph, the boarder, had told my patient that if she ever went to Rheinfelden, where they had a huge bakery specialising in luxury high-class cakes, his family would give her, free, the holiday of a lifetime.

When we had said that we had planned to go by car through Europe, and she was welcome to travel with us, paying only the crossing fare of three pounds, her face lit up. Her back pain got less and she wrote to Joseph, who had by then gone home, telling him the news.

When holiday time came, we picked up the excited lady very late at night. I had worked twelve hours that day, but it was no trouble driving to Dover. I slept a little on the boat, and drove to Switzerland, which was about three hundred miles, where my wife and I had booked into a hotel for the night.

We were delighted when the bakery and their outdoor café were right on the River Rhine and had a landing for many of the tourist ships. The people getting off the ships scoffed all manner of scrumptious cream cakes etc.

Joseph said he would take his guest to Calais in two weeks' time. That gave us time to drive through Europe and meet on the appointed day at the right time.

When we did pick her up, she couldn't stop talking about her marvellous holiday, and it added to her joy to see her delight. Some time later, the manager of the bakery that Joseph went to, came to me for treatment every Friday at eight in the morning so that he could be at his office before nine.

CHAPTER 25

QUESTIONS AND ANSWERS

Doctor Albert you don't give much credit to the medical profession.

Albert I think the medics and hospitals do a wonderful job but tell me why doctors are so unhealthy.

Doctor What would you have us do?

Albert Press for more prevention and start checking everybody the same, but I want you to make allowances for different sizes and ages.

Doctor We already do this.

Albert Not really, you can't say that when I know that you often give 10^{cc} of an injection to a slim girl of sixteen and give the same dose to a forty-year-old man who weighs twenty stone. Also, what about the drugs being too strong?

Doctor What strong drugs? They come to us tried and tested.

Albert I think with some you should try half the dose until you're sure.

Doctor What would you do with anti-inflamatory capsules?

Albert There are plenty of substitutes, and remember forty per cent of drugs that you prescribe for people are thrown away.

Doctor Come off it Albert, you're going over the top.

Albert No Sir, I'm quoting the *Medical Journal*.

Doctor You have no concept of the strain we work in.

Albert I give you that, but if you got fitter you may be able to cope with the strain better.

Doctor How the hell can we find time to get fitter?

Albert Follow the natural rules in my first book and tell your patients that drugs can not make real health and they must do something to help themselves.

Doctor What about the wonderful operations and the replacement of organs which has given many people a much better life?

Albert I most definitely approve of this but a famous professor said that the finest doctors are air, water and the sun.

Doctor What the devil do we do about that?

Albert Well now the air is badly polluted, water is going less and the sun is stronger and more dangerous.

Doctor So again what do we do about this?

Albert PRAY.

Good Night and God Bless You All.

CHAPTER 26

PROFESSIONAL WRESTLING

I was privileged to be in the dressing room at one of the first professional wrestling shows in Britain, at Bradford's Manningham Hall. This was organised by the splendid Health and Strength Club — The Manningham All Rounders. It was certainly an eye-opener; the wrestlers were very fit, young and beautifully-built athletes. Some of them were tumblers and acrobats. It was a change from the rather slower amateur wrestling, and it caught the eighty per cent female audience, who screamed their delight at this new entertainment.

It was not long before I was treating many of these tough lads; most of them had a great sense of humour and this encouraged the audience, who sometimes joined in the fun!

At Kelvin Hall in Glasgow, an irate lady dashed into the ring, pulled a large hatpin out of her hat and stabbed it right through Peter Cecil Knowles Hugh's calf muscle — left sticking out inches on both sides.

Another lady belted a very big wrestler with her strong stick, breaking it on his head. These happenings, and some comical in the ring, made for an exciting night.

When the World Heavyweight Champion came from Canada to Manchester, he was brought to me by eighteen-stone Basil Goldstone, a friend who I had treated many times. The champ introduced himself — "I am Carl Von Warden. In America I twist de back, I go to one man, click, he put it right. The next day I wrestle in Manchester,

I twist de back,'' — using his fingers to emphasise — ''I go to one, I go to two, I go to three, damn it, I go to five men. Nobody can put it right. Can you?''

Looking at the terrific spinal muscles in total spasm on one side, I was rather doubtful unless I could lay him out first. He was twice as big as me and looked ready to eat me. I persuaded him to get on the couch and gave him a long session of infrared heat hoping to relax him. Then put him twisted on the couch with one leg hanging off. I got Basil to sit on his shoulder whilst I jumped my eleven stone on his raised hip thus suddenly turning Carl's spine away from the locked fifth lumbar vertebra. There was suddenly a sharp crack — the victim jumped off the couch saying ''It is right I know, I wrestle tomorrow.'' And so he did.

It was a dangerous manoeuvre, not to be tried again, but after nearly shaking my hand off, he eventually left at just midnight.

Peter Gisburg, an antique specialist in Manchester, was wrestling in a bull ring at Alicante in Spain. He didn't like the dirty tricks the Spanish local champion did in the first round. His tricks started again in the second round, so Peter laid the Spaniard out cold, to the consternation of the audience. Peter then made an almost deadly mistake — he stood up raised his hands to the side of his head and pretended to be a bull. The crowd rushed the ring and Peter had to fight his way to the dressing room; he was in rather a bad way, one arm cut to the bone from shoulder to elbow, also bleeding in other places. The police managed to keep the Spanish out of the door and got an ambulance which took Peter to the local hospital. At the hospital they threw him on a trolley and left him to bleed. Despite Peter's shouts, nobody came for a long time and then he was treated like a vandal — the doctor roughly stitched him up without any painkillers at all. After this the police charged him thirty pounds for causing a riot, thirty pounds for the ambulance and another thirty for the doctor. Peter got himself into more trouble as the poor lad could not drive his car, so he took a flight home to Manchester Hospital where the staff couldn't believe that a doctor had done the terrible stitching. Someone suggested it was the decorator who was working in the hospital.

Peter now lives quietly on farmland in lovely Cheshire.

BOBBY STEELE

This wonderful athlete certainly had a full life working on real manual jobs and wrestling abroad as well as in Britain. He worked the Canadian pipelines to San Francisco and also worked in Mexico for three years. He was always training and wrestling. Bobby toured Spain for four months with a group of wrestlers.

Back in the UK, Bobby tells of wrestling in a London tournament when, on the first night he sustained a severe neck injury. He drove all night to Oldham to see me and wrestled back in London the next day.

Bobby was a tough lad, which probably saved his life years later when he ran a garage in a rough area of Manchester. The following event happened in January 1989. His staff had left; Bobby was checking up when two masked men, one armed with a club, the other with a machete, dashed in and knocked Bobby to the ground. The first blow was aimed at Bobby's head; he flung his arm to stop the machete splitting his head and received severe wounds in his forearm. The next blow almost severed his kneecap. One blow even lashed his face. However they didn't know who their opponent was and Bobby managed to get up and threw one of them through the door. He smashed the other one and rolled him down the garage forecourt. The two men got away, but Bobby was in hospital for quite a while. His description got them later when they used a gun on someone, and finally got jailed for ten years each.

Bobby was only five foot six inches high, but nearly as wide, and still a great lad.

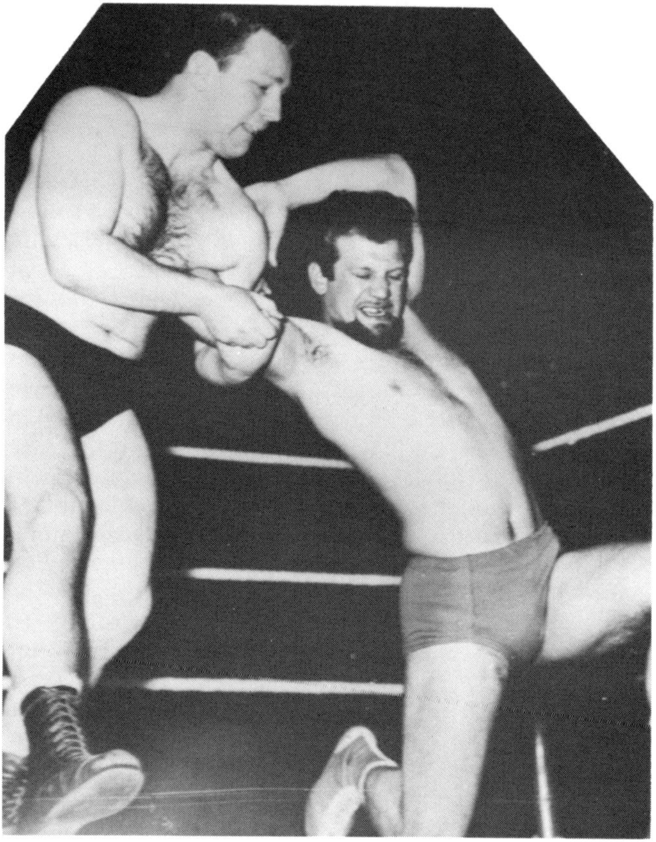

Bobby Steele and Peter Gisburg

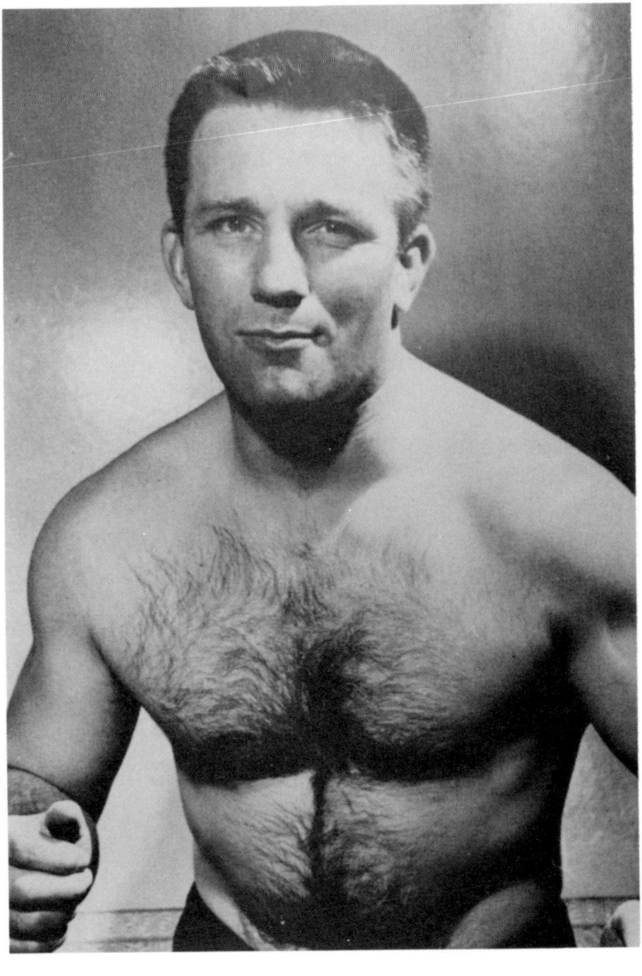

Bobby Steele — A Man of Iron

FRANCIS ST CLAIR GREGORY

Francis St Clair Gregory was Amateur Heavyweight Champion of Cornwall at Cornish Wrestling when he was eighteen years old. He came up North, played a forward in Rugby League for St Helens Rugby Club and started professional wrestling. His two fine lads became pro wrestlers. It was many years before he came to me and I was appalled at his condition — sixteen stone and full of arthritis.

"When did you finish wrestling Francis?" I asked.

"Oh, I am wrestling in Aberdeen in two days' time."

This I could hardly believe, so I gave him the best advice that I could. "If you get caught in a neck lock, just give in — if you try to throw out of it, your arthritic neck could break."

Francis was a gentle giant and a perfect gentleman — I was sure he would never hurt anyone intentionally but he must have been suffering for years — every joint was nearly solid with arthritis. There is no doubt in my mind that many of these brave entertainers suffered, became crippled and a few died, because of the knocks and falls in tough wrestling.

Francis bought a villa in Spain hoping the sun would help, but a few years later he came home and died. He was a wonderful, kind and courageous gentleman.

Another colourful character came to me in great pain; this was a Rochdale man, Johnny Eagles; he had a large coloured eagle tattooed across his broad chest. On his way home from fighting in Aberdeen, Johnny came motoring round a stiff bend in the dark and ran slap into an articulated lorry which was jackknifed right across the road. With no chance of stopping, Johnny hung on, bending the steering wheel. He refused to go to hospital and just managed to get to my clinic, where it was obvious that both shoulders were dislocated. No way would he go to hospital, although I told him it would be very painful to

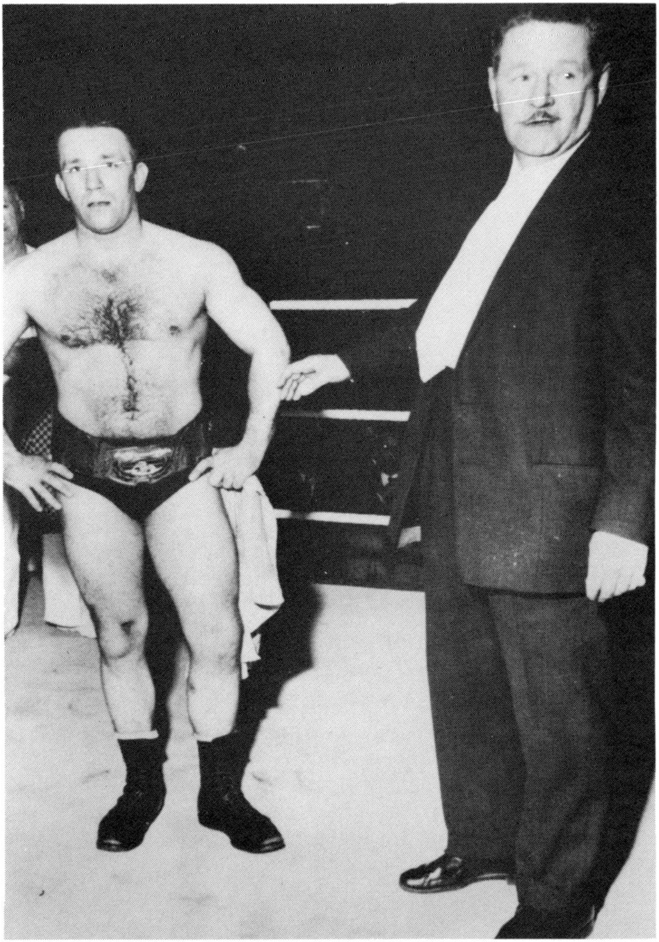

Bobby Steele and George De Relwykow — Promoter

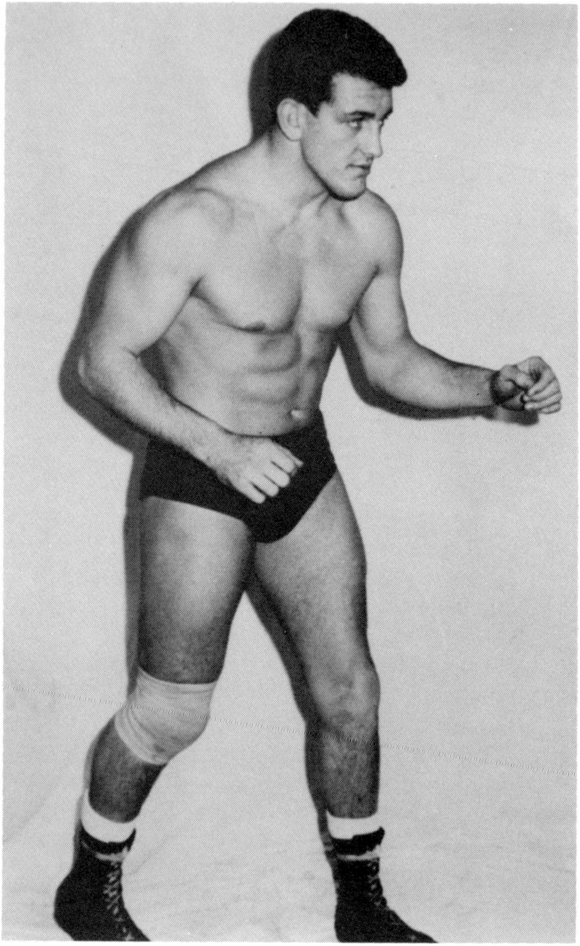

Bill Robinson, 18-stone Manchester Wrestler

manipulate without anaesthetic. I knew the pain because I had previously had one shoulder dislocated. However there was no moaning from Johnny as I forced the joints, using my leg and foot for leverage. I made both of us a drink; I think it was me that really needed one. I told him that his wrestling was over for about six weeks. Two weeks later I was watching the wrestling on television and there he was performing with strapping on both shoulders. He later wrestled in Japan and California, and is now in the motor industry in Seattle, Washington, USA.

BILL ROBINSON

A great character, was six foot three inches and eighteen stone. His name was Bill Robinson of Manchester and he was an early member of Failsworth Lads Club, which was helped by a wealthy patient of mine — Mr Stanley Butters. Bill's father was a noted boxer, but Bill only had sight in one eye through damage in childhood, so it was wrestling for him. He carried the British flag everywhere he went and in Japan he really scared the natives walking about the streets draped in the Union Jack. In America he was attacked by a gang wielding iron bars. He is now a security guard in Las Vegas.

Scores of these tough lads passed through my hands and it was a pleasure to do what I could for them. I consider it was a great privilege to have known them.

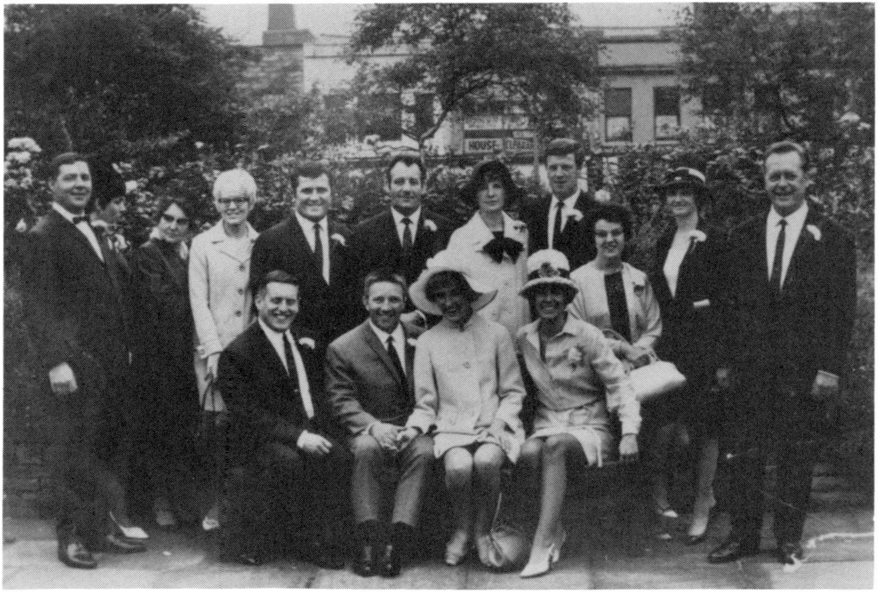

Bobby Steele's Wedding
Pictured here with his wrestling pals

CHAPTER 27

A FEW PATIENTS AND A DETECTIVE

The amazing Mr Graham Brock is my next subject in this book. I must record what this man has done in the thirty-four years of his life. His mother, who has been a patient of mine for a long time, brought him to me to see if he could benefit from my treatment; he was seventeen, six foot tall and six and a half stone in weight. The boy had a very bad case of anorexia.

When his mother brought him she was in floods of tears and said that she couldn't do anything with him.

I first gave him a relaxing massage — talking to him all the time. I gave him a few treatments with me only massaging him and he started to listen to what I was saying and took an interest in the photos of well-developed men.

Within a month of me treating him, Graham was doing light training and then went on to body building. He was actually sprouting muscles, where before there was only skin and bone.

In five years he was a well-built twelve-stone man, enjoyed life and had a great appetite.

Mr Brock started running and completed his first marathon in 1986 when he was twenty-three years old. In a fairly short time, he had also completed thirty half-marathons. He did them all for charity. He also finished two triathalons which entailed him to do a severe swim, then forty miles cycling, finishing with a full marathon.

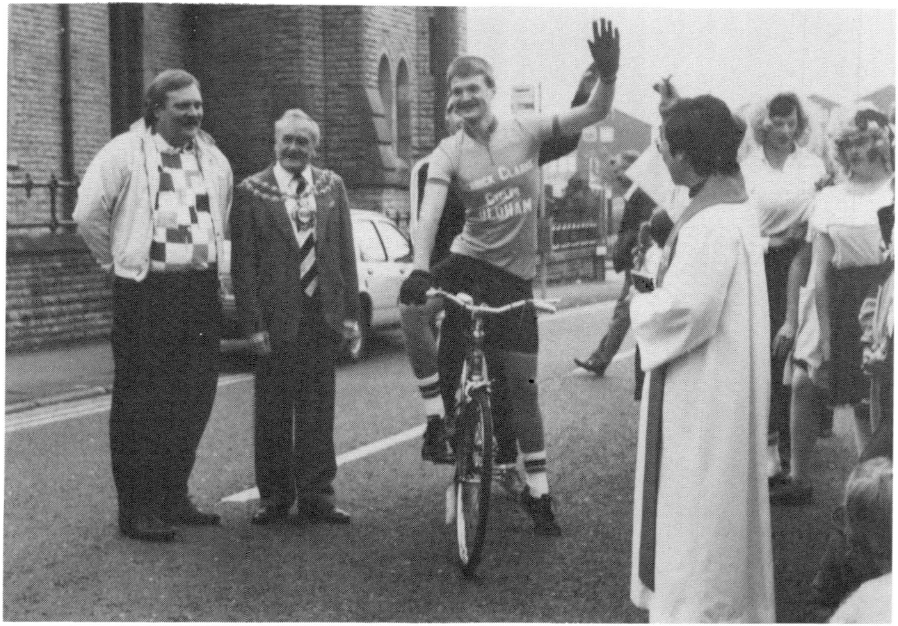

Graham Brock

Graham really enjoyed cycling and turned to do long distance cycling. He managed to do a cycle from John o'Groat's to Land's End in nine and a half days. In the picture he had just finished cycling to Blackpool and back with a blind man on the back of the tandem. He did this again for charity.

Mr Brock did nine years as a policeman and today holds down a position as an Engineer Inspector in coaches and buses.

I feel really proud of his achievements and am honoured to have helped this great man become what he is. Not everyone can rise to such a great height, and quite a few tend to give up when the going gets tough, but there is something in having a go. As the body improves with sensible exercise, so does the mind; the circulation improves and the body's natural healing properties are awakened. The human physique is unique in that it always strives to improve, providing that it gets a reasonable diet and enough exercise.

If you are worried, depressed or upset, the answer is not to rest but get up and GO.

In my kind of work, one sometimes has to use strength as well as skill, and in a small number of cases it hurts just as we can be hurt by the dentist or chiropodist. It is usual to tell some people that we don't hurt unnecessarily and our only thought is to cure or at least alleviate. In all my sixty-two years of work I have had very seldom any complaints, but one incident caused me some worry.

A man came to me with lower back pain. This complaint was very common and was usually caused by bad posture and an exceptionally hollow lumbar spine. I have treated hundreds of these cases and for sometime I have given only one treatment and then told them to do the exercises, that I had told them about, for a couple of months after the treatment. This usually finished the job.

To start off with I gave him infrared heat, a massage,

manipulation and showed him the necessary exercises. I told him to keep the exercises up for six months. I also told him like every new patient, that if they got more pain or they got worried, that they must come back to me or give me a ring.

I heard no news from this particular gentleman for six months. When the sixth month had arrived, his wife rang me and told me that they had got a solicitor to take me to Court because her husband was in pain and hadn't been able to work since he had seen me. I asked her address and as soon as I had finished work for the day I went round to their house and was knocking on their door.

A little girl opened the door and I dashed in to find the man sitting almost on top of the television and in his dressing gown. I told the man to get up and touch his toes. He refused to do this nor any other exercise I asked him to do. That was all I wanted to know and I told him that the final part of my treatment was up to him to do the exercises but if he hadn't done them then it was his fault, that he hasn't got any better. His next remark was that he had seven kids and the solicitor wouldn't cost him anything.

When I got back home I was quite happy with what I had found and the situation that I was in.

The next morning I received a letter in the post from his solicitor. I was furious with the wording in the letter. The letter said:

> 'We are instructed that the severe back condition which our client developed resulted in negligent or inappropriate treatment on your behalf, and we are to pursue a claim against you for damages. Please refer this matter to your insurers and ask them to contact us at once.'

The so-called victim also claimed that he was given severe exercises, but the exercises he was given were really quite simple exercises like bending down on a low stool as shown in my previous book, *Self Help and Movement for*

Rheumatic Sufferers; published by Stockwell, Ilfracombe. Many hundreds of my patients have done these exercises and still do the exercise to keep the lumbar discs and the spinal vertebrae supple.

Due to the almost certainty of the man with seven children getting legal aid, I ignored the solicitors and decided to get myself a solicitor. I rang our local judge, John Lord, who first thanked me for the work that I did on his mother. He told me that she thought the world of me; this made me very pleased with myself and made me feel slightly happier about the case. He told me to see a good solicitor whom he admired very much and I also had to tell him that Mr Lord was also interested in the case.

The first time I went to see the solicitor, I took along my book which showed the exercise I had given the man quite clearly.

Someone started to spread the news that I was in trouble and within three weeks I had letters from scores of people, mainly present or ex-patients. Lord Langford wrote from Wales, and Lord Crawshaw wrote from the House of Lords; Ex-Chief Constable of Oldham, Mr Fred Berry wrote his support from Liverpool and I even got lots of support from Ireland, in the certain knowledge that I was ready to go to Court.

At that time I and three solicitors coming for treatment, and one told me to tread carefully, he said "I am certain you can't lose but even winning could cost you a few thousands of pounds. No judge would order the costs of Court to a man with seven children, so you would have to pay his costs."

This staggered me so I took the advice of Lord Crawford and got myself a detective. The late Lord Crawshaw OBE, TD, DL, MP, World Champion Walker, had been a patient of mine and had bought and paid for quite a few patients from the Liverpool area.

The detective recommended by ex-Sergeant Allcock of Oldham Police was the ex-Chief Superintendent of the

Manchester Police, Allan Robinson, who after retiring, started a detective agency in Rochdale.

Earlier, during the war, he had worked with my dear wife at a local confectioners, and at one time had been one of my club lads at the Health and Strength Club.

At once Allan came to see us and put our minds at rest. He told us that in one month he would know everything about the 'Chappy'. He kept his promise and within a month had found out lots about the man. Although the man claimed he had not been able to work after my treatment, Allan had discovered that he had not worked for a while before I had given him treatment. He did have a fairly good lifestyle and drove a smart car.

Not long before the case Allan made an appointment to see my solicitor, and put his facts on the table. Sometime after the claimant left his double council house and that was the end. I paid my solicitor and wanted to pay Allan, but he refused to accept his fee.

May I now print another one of the letters that I got in this time of trouble.

HOUSING UNITS OF HOLLINWOOD

JANUARY 1986

TO WHOM IT MAY CONCERN

Mr Byram has given treatment to myself and my family over a considerable number of years. He has also treated colleagues and friends whom I have recommended should attend his rooms — people who have had particular problems. Many of whom have been given relief from persistent complaints after their visits.

I along with thousands of other patients, who have had the privilege, and been fortunate to receive treatment, endorse the exceptional service which Mr Byram has given.

It is also his philosophy that clients can help themselves, before and after treatment, well explained and illustrated in his own publication, combining common sense with exercise — a book proved most helpful to many sufferers.

There can be no question as to his ability and desire to help those generally in pain.

J. H. PELLOWE.

(I treated his father in 1935.)

CHAPTER 28

EATING AND FASTING

Almost everyone knows that the human body requires both food and drink, but some don't know when to stop. Please I ask you all EAT to LIVE don't LIVE to EAT. I know it is one of life's pleasures to eat, but it is also one of life's disasters to overeat. Remember, the stomach is the body's powerhouse; overfill it and the whole body suffers.

After twenty-five years of age, the body has stopped growing taller, but if it gets too much food and drink it usually keeps growing, but dangerously outwards.

Most definitely after twenty-five you don't require half as much sustenance as you did when you were younger. That is unless you are using far more energy. By this I mean physical energy, heavy work, training, playing vigorous sports, body building, cycling or marathon running. If you do this, then you can indulge a little more. In recent years there has been a fad for drinking more water; some stupid slimming diets even advocate drinking up to ten glasses of water daily. Of course this could slim a person by making him or her ill, thereby losing weight, due to two things; firstly by overspeeding digestion and washing away the vitamins and minerals of the system; second, by washing away the wonderful slimy coating that covers and protects the alimentary canal.

Over sixty years ago, at the Westwood Health and Strength Club, a few enthusiasts and I, experimented by cutting down on all fluids, even though we trained hard. As we got to less than one pint of fluid each day, everyone felt fitter than ever before. This was certainly against medical opinion, but to this day I restrict my fluids to less than one and a half pints of fluids, and I still exercise. Surely the medics know that there is over eighty per cent water in potatoes, bread, salads and most fruit. Perhaps many folk don't want to go to my length, and I can't blame them, but if you want to feel really good as you grow older, you must eat and drink a little less, and keep up some daily exercise — even if it only means walking two miles a day.

Another aid to better health is an occasional fast to give the stomach a well-deserved rest. Whilst at first one should be most careful, don't fast while growing, don't fast in cold weather, don't fast if you are anaemic, or if suffering an active disease. One should only fast by cutting down on food over a few days, then start a complete fast for one day taking only water. The beginning of food should be very light, easily digested, and then start on an improved diet. Later you could try two days; often any pain that you had before, will be much easier. Longer fasts should only be done under supervision. When the body is deprived of food, the organs of digestion have a well-needed rest, and the body lives on its reserves and some fat; thus cleaning itself. In long fasts I found a remarkable sign to prevent a long fast turning in to starving. After two or three days without food, the tongue becomes badly coated, which shows the amount of waste in the body. The more coated the tongue is, the cleansing property of the body shows up clearly. As the tongue starts to clear up, it indicates that the body has started to do its own spring-clean. At first the outer edge of the tongue reverts back to its natural red colour, and slowly this spreads all over. This would take a long time in an unfit body and it would require careful watching. The fast must stop before all the tongue is red. It always starts outwards and when it gets near the centre, it's time to stop, because any longer and we would not be fasting but starving.

As I have said, don't do a long fast without supervision. Many times I have fasted for a whole week, with great benefit, not only feeling fitter physically, but mentally fitter and calmer. I think one of the greatest long-term benefits of fasting is the reduction of the stored sugar in the liver. When you stop sugar and carbohydrates, the liver responds by pumping its often overload of sugar into the bloodstream to be used up.

RELAXATION

Total relaxation is not possible. There are internal muscles, organs and secretions that are not under our conscious control, but by learning a better awareness of our external muscles and concentrating on these, we can all improve our relaxation.

Basically there are only two exercises, concentration and relaxation. If you can concentrate by tightening one, or a group of muscles — shutting out the mind — then let go, the muscle should flop like jelly. Only by tightening first can one afterwards get the desired looseness.

Practise this in bed when it is difficult to sleep: Try to tighten the closed eyes. Tighten the neck, the fists, then the whole body and don't forget about your feet, screwing up your toes. Hold this position for thirty seconds, then flop trying to let everything go, at the same time, concentrating on ONE simple thought in the mind — breathing to a count. On one breathe in, and on two breathe out — it won't work if the mind is busy thinking about what is for breakfast. It is not really possible to think of food and work and fall asleep. So put one simple thought into your mind, instead of the usual complication. It is almost impossible to think of nothing and counting sheep is not as good as counting breaths — and I don't mean just counting numbers in and out.

Next day, try the muscles; sit down, lift your right arm straight out in front of you; put two fingers of your left hand under right wrist, holding the weight of your right arm. Quickly move the fingers away and very often the arm is still out in front; when if it was relaxed, it should have fallen down by its weight and gravity. You will find it relaxes better if you stiffen the arm first; then it will fall easier and be limp at your side. With help you can do the legs; by getting your partner to put a hand under your leg (lying supine), which should be straight and raised about six inches off the floor, as the hand is suddenly removed the leg should almost crash down. Lift the shoulders as high as possible, hold for a few seconds, then flop.

Sit on a kitchen table and try to relax almost as though your body is falling through the table. Legs over the edge and alternative swinging loosely about one foot in front; then the same under the table. Rest your hands on your thighs, get an easy pendulum movement with hardly any effort. Four minutes of this will often relax the lower back and in many cases ease a painful one. Pain is always increased by the mind and if we are worried we create a chemical imbalance causing the suprarenal glands to secrete adrenaline into the bloodstream. Adrenaline is acid, a powerful stimulant and a poison. As with everything in the body, it has a purpose; when we are angry, depressed, frustrated or in danger, adrenaline gives us extra strength to fight our way out of the situation; but beware of leaving a residue in the body. Don't just sit down shaking with fury or whatever, get up and use physical energy to use up the powerful acid — if left in the bloodstream it will certainly cause trouble.

CHAPTER 29

ARTHUR LEES, MBE

Amongst many of my pain-suffering patients, I must pay tribute to this person. I knew Arthur when he was a young smart lad; he lived close to me and certainly a healthy teenager and a good cricketer.

In 1935, when I got married and moved from the district, I lost touch. In 1960 I still recognised him when he passed our house in an invalid car. I asked my dear wife to stop him if he came back back. With some difficulty we got him inside, and I got the full story of his troubles. His whole spine was completely solid with ankylosing spondylitis — from head to tail every vertebra had grown into the next, thereby fusing the spinal column. His arms were not too bad, but his legs were pretty hopeless and he was hardly able to sit down. From that day on I gave him some treatment on both his ankles, which helped him to negotiate steps much better.

The spinal trouble was obviously caused by him being encased in plaster for over two years. This appalled me and I certainly felt very sorry for him undergoing this treatment.

Mr Lees was the Honorary Secretary of the local Inskip League of Friendship and because sitting was most difficult, he stood all day typing. He along with seven others (five in wheelchairs), had started the League in 1949, and later by hard work and good organisation had got a social centre built in Oldham, 1955. This was opened

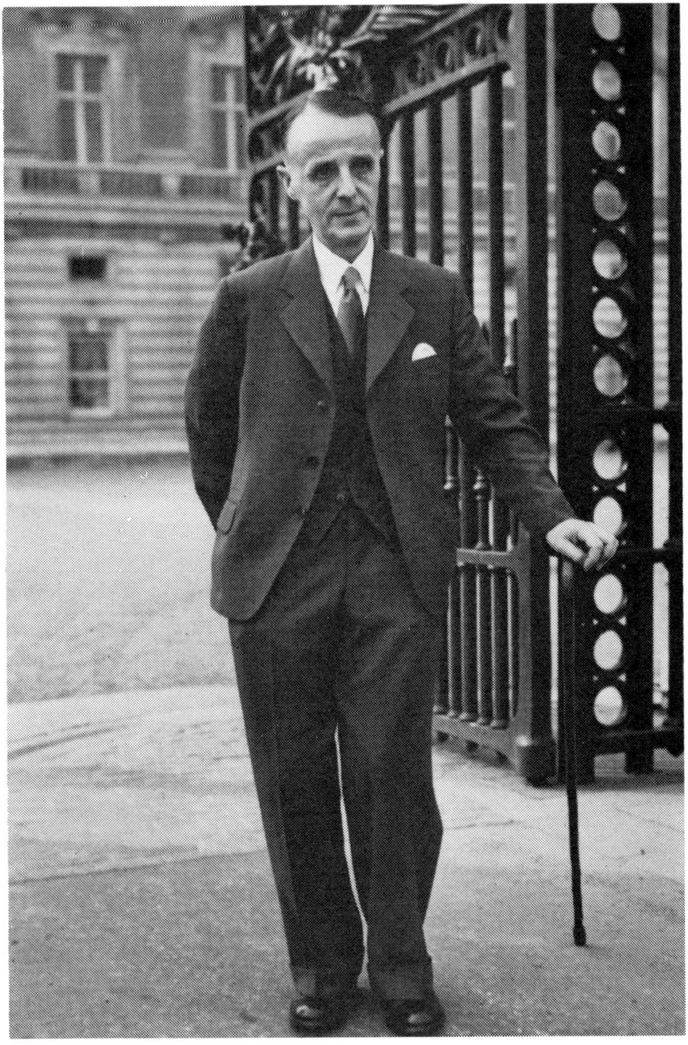

Arthur Lees, MBE (At the Palace)

by Wilfred Pickles, OBE and the Mayor of Oldham, Alderman H. H. Webster, JP, whose wife was a patient of mine, and also my next-door neighbour.

A general invitation was open to any disabled to join at one shilling per year.

Before the building began, they had five hundred members and three hundred associates; the Inskip League was also spreading to many other towns around Britain. Backed by Oldham Council and registered with the National Assistance Act, 1948, the centre became a haven for many people. They organised concerts, parties, table tennis competitions, outings and billiards. After years of working at the centre, Arthur was honoured by the Queen, but not long after tragedy struck.

When Arthur was coming home from Blackpool in his invalid car, a man who was driving a lorry, shot across the road and smashed into Arthur and killed the poor man. Arthur's friend, who had been driving in another car, just watched in horror. The man, who had been drinking, got nine months in jail. Arthur's dear wife, now eighty-eight, has been widowed for nearly forty years.

CHAPTER 30

MY SPARRING PARTNER

My acrobatic partner married shortly after Nan and I; his wife Emily (formerly Livesy) now Heathcote, had a small shop near the club and was very interested in all the club's activities and often came to watch the Warwick Bros.

She was a strong healthy girl and gave Harry four healthy children, and today at eighty-eight, looks back at some of the many exploits of the Westwood Health and Strength Club.

By hard training, Harry and I established a good rapport and could almost tell what each other was thinking. He was a strong, healthy young man and never let me down, although we often tried quite dangerous stunts in practise. It was a great sorrow when Harry came home from work and suddenly died before Emily could do anything. This was a mystery, but I think I know the cause, although I never mentioned it at the sad time. Some years before Harry had been injured when a fall of timber crashed onto his leg leaving a bad gash. This didn't heal very well, despite visiting a specialist and left a darkish scar. I really think that the day he died he probably knocked this leg, disturbed a clot in the scar, which finished in the poor man's heart.

A great sorrow to us all, Harry was just forty-five years old.

CHAPTER 31

NAN

You have read in an earlier chapter about my wife's emphysema, mainly due to working in a cotton mill from fourteen to nineteen years of age. Because I couldn't have done much without her, I want to tell you how we got together.

With my interest in hand balancing, health, studying the body, vegetarianism, treating people and training at the club, I hadn't much time for girls, dancing or the cinema — in fact, I must have been a real crank. At twenty-four I took an interest in Nan. I saw a rather poorly girl with a terrible cough, but she had a lovely smile and a great character. After leaving the factory she worked in a confectionary shop. Mostly from eight a.m. to eight p.m. for one pound each week. When we first started courting (only two nights each week), I always went to the gym first — must not miss any training. When she got pneumonia, something stirred in me because of the way she smilingly fought the infection. This I think started my real love for Nan. She was always interested in everything I did, and even endured my pet treatment for her bad cough — equal parts of black treacle and mustard, well mixed with a tiny amount of water. This usually stopped any cough, but it was horrible and almost burnt the throat. We married in 1935 when I was twenty-five years old and my Nan was a great partner. Although we were deprived of children, it was I know, a sore point to Nan, who loved all children; but as always, I never heard her grumble. When I was in full practice at home, she was a tower of strength to me and delighted when I had children in for treatment. She could put any child at ease in a few minutes. We lived together, worked together, had holidays together, and were together twenty-four hours each day. Some people may get tired of seeing each other all day, but I can say that it only strengthened our love. Even though Nan was ill, we still had great holidays. I want to record one such holiday.

Doctor Gordon Fletcher and his family came to live next door to us and we soon became friends. Three boys and lovely Sarah, who at the age of two, became most friendly with Nan, who was enchanted with the bonny girl. Every morning we heard this call, "Mrs Byram can I come in?" Sure, and she was in most of the day including her nightly bath. She was no trouble and Nan really loved her to be near. This led to one of our best holidays. One day Sarah said I am going on holiday to Australia, but her mother, Lorna told us that they were emigrating. This certainly devastated Nan — it was like losing one of our own, even if we had one. Dr Fletcher had been given a good position there, with first-class travel by sea, including his furniture and car, all at the Australian's expense. Nan couldn't face seeing them go, so we dashed off to the caravan in Wales. She was so upset that I told her that we would go there on our next holiday. I booked early and paid; got the air tickets and then Britain devalued and called on me for another four hundred pounds, despite the fact that we had already paid in full. We had a taxi to Ringwood Airport, then first stop New York; off the plane and a fine meal in the airport café. Next stop San Francisco, for six hours' sightseeing. We then called at Honolulu and on to Fiji for a wonderful week at a rather nice hotel, where we had lots of fun with the laughing carefree Fijians. Then down to Sydney where our friend Doctor Fletcher picked us up to travel a hundred miles north to Williamstown — a training airstrip, teaching pilots to fly French Mirage fighter planes. Gordon was the medical officer at this very secure unit and the training was I think for a possible engagement in the then Vietnamese War. It was great to see our friends who really were homesick and the welcome was marvellous. Gordon had arranged a deep-sea fishing trip in my honour — what a great idea — but a little doubt crept in when the thirty-foot boat shook us all up going through thirty-foot breakers. Two of the party were sick and never got up from the bottom of the boat all day. However, when we started to catch good fish, most of the British on board enjoyed a smashing time. After getting back on land, we found that we were still sailing, we couldn't balance and we could hardly walk. It took two days to really recover. We did most of the usual trips, Blue Mountains and the nerve-testing drive over Sydney Bridge at peak time.

I had a patient at home whose brother lived in Sydney; this patient hadn't seen his brother for twenty years and wondered if we might see him. A tall order, but Nan and I flew down to Sydney, sailed across Sydney Harbour and found the address. He and his wife were delighted, and after a nice meal took us round the sights, including the famous Manley Beach. A great day out, which they appeared to enjoy as much as we did.

Nearly three weeks gone in a flash and it was time to sorryfully leave the Fletchers and fly home. The eldest boy Nigel wanted to come home with us; said he could live with Uncle Charlie. However Gordon had only signed for four years and though the Australians had tried hard to keep him, he decided Blighty was calling; more particularly his wife Lorna, who wasn't keen on the thousands of flies etc.

Lorna and the children flew home as soon as the four years had finished, but Gordon still had a little work to do. Nan and I drove to Heathrow Airport, picked them up, drove home, and squeezed them in for the night. We then went house hunting for them. When Gordon got home he found a position on Oldham Health and later became a Medical Officer to Merseyside.

Despite Nan's health, we nearly always managed holidays at the caravan in North Wales and also abroad.

Once in the Algarve, Portugal, we arrived late at night and next morning Nan got up early suffering from gastroenteritis; it was easy to diagnose because she had had it before. We got the local doctor, who was a friend, who told us that we had brought it from England, but later we found there was quite an epidemic around and the doctor's wife had been in bed with it for two weeks. He gave us tablets and told me he was hopelessly busy and that we had to try and manage on our own. The tablets were useless because Nan was sick all the time — so next morning I went to his packed surgery asking for injections. He told me that he couldn't possibly come but I did not bother because I informed him that I would give the injections to her myself each day. He gave me the injections and told me to ring him at ten in the morning and six each evening to report on Nan's condition. Nan was very rough for eight days, then I slowly saw an improvement and by the time we got home she was OK. The Travel Club of Great Britain, which we had used a number of times, offered us a free extra week if we would stay, but Nan, as always, wanted to get home now she was fit to travel.

Nan had been on steroids for years, and the side effects were damaging her skin. The slightest knock opened the skin and caused bruising and often bleeding. Some of these took months to heal.

In later years, my niece, next of kin, and her husband, bought a hotel in Cornwall, on the coast near Bude. We were invited any time we liked, and after a pleasant three hundred mile drive down — which Nan stood very well — we enjoyed Cornwall immensely. The second time we had to cut the visit short as Nan's right leg suddenly lost colour and became rather cold. I couldn't even find a pulse in the groin. So we drove home quickly and got to our splendid Dr MacKenzie in less than five hours. He knew the right consultant at Oldham Hospital and it was soon cleared.

We had another trip to Cornwall and poor Nan got gastroenteritis again on the second day of our visit. Two local doctors attended to her whilst she was still in bed, and two days later when the vomiting had stopped, Nan wanted to go home. She was still rather poorly, but because I drove steadily, we made it back. I sent Nan straight to bed. Dr MacKenzie did his magic and in three days Nan was up, still smiling.

The last time we went to Portugal, Nan was forced to have a wheelchair, which she didn't like, so she said never again; we will now look back at the good times we have had.

At the age of eighty-three, I decided to completely retire because it was obvious that Nan was getting weaker. Some months later, whilst we were at the caravan, Nan stubbed her left big toe. We couldn't stop the bleeding so I drove her to Glanclwyd Hospital in Rhyl at midnight, where they kindly and professionally did a good job. Back home the healing flesh had caused an ingrowing toenail. This became inflamed and was starting to go black. A wonderful chiropodist, Mrs Cheshire, came to the house. We told her that a year ago in Cornwall a doctor told us that the toe would have been better if it had been taken off. Mrs Cheshire agreed and said that she would remove the toe within two months. After working on the toe every night for seven weeks she took the toe off leaving the joint perfect — almost a miracle. This was completed with Nan sat on the settee, no moaning and no tears — as it was years before — when she had suffered terribly with Ménière's disease and tinnitus. Her balance had gone and if she closed her eyes she would fall to the ground and then become dreadfully sick. She would often sit for ages with a bowl between her knees and I hardly ever heard her complain.

In 1994, my dear wife was feeling much weaker, but if anyone asked her it was always "I'm all right." Her right foot was cold and causing some pain, which made me think back to when we rushed back from Cornwall with a possible stoppage in the circulation in the same leg.

I soon got our good Dr MacKenzie to come and he asked Dr Mackintosh, the top surgeon at the Royal Oldham Hospital, to visit us. The next day they came together and Dr Mackintosh said that the leg needed to be amputated, not just above the foot as I expected, but well above the knee. Within two days they sent for Nan and after a couple of delays she was in theatre. One hour after the operation Nan was sitting up in bed reading the *Oldham Chronicle* and looking real good. The staff couldn't stop looking at her and nobody could believe that she was eighty-three years of age.

Three days later she picked up an infection and was laid low. The specialist told me she would be better away from the many bugs that invaded the surgical wards, and suggested Total Care — which was only a mile away. I managed to fix this with their Matron and Nan was in a private room. This only lasted one week and then I thought my pal was dying, and the Matron agreed when I told her that I wanted to take Nan home. She had always said she wanted to die before me, wanted to die at home and wanted to give her eyes to the Eye Hospital in Manchester. As I got her home, my niece Christina, had just arrived from Cornwall. She was a tower of strength for the next three days, supported by our fine doctor and the excellent District Nurses that came twice daily.

Nan was in great pain and we gave her morphine every two hours, but nothing lessened the terrible pain. I had asked why both her arms were bandaged from wrist to shoulder, and now I saw the answer — blood was seeping through the bandages.

We could understand that steroids had killed her, but they certainly had kept her alive for perhaps twenty years.

Three days and nights at home, and my true love passed away on the twenty-ninth of July 1994. Her eyes went straight to the hospital and her body was cremated.

There were very many people and friends at the church and I shall be ever indebted to the Reverend Hunper, whose lovely sermon and talk really stirred something in me.

My life is not as lonely as I had expected, I feel Nan's presence at all times and I talk to her every day — Thanking her for a lovely fifty-nine years of happiness.

TOMORROW IS COMING
THE POSSIBILITIES ARE ENDLESS

ALBERT